Essential Exercises for the Childbearing Year

Essential Exercises for the Childbearing Year

A Guide to Health and Comfort Before and After Your Baby Is Born

by Elizabeth Noble, R.P.T.

Illustrations by Maya M. Jacob

Foreword by Emanuel A. Friedman, M.D.

Preface to the Second Edition by Doris Haire, D.M.S.

SECOND EDITION, REVISED

Houghton Mifflin Company   Boston

To Geoff

Book design by Dianne Smith, Designworks, Inc.

Library of Congress Cataloging in Publication Data

Noble, Elizabeth, date.
    Essential exercises for the childbearing year.

    Bibliography: p.
    Includes index.
    1. Pregnancy.   2. Exercise for women.   3. Prenatal
care.   4. Postnatal care.   I. Title.
RG558.7.N62   1981   618.2′4   81-2685
ISBN 0-395-31561-1   AACR2
ISBN 0-395-31543-3 (pbk.)
Printed in the United States of America
AL 10 9 8 7 6 5 4

Contents

Acknowledgments

I am grateful to innumerable people, childbearers and colleagues, in both the United States and Australia, who shared their feelings and observations with me over the years. In particular I wish to mention Margaret D. Verco, Director of Physiotherapy, Queen Victoria Hospital for Women, Adelaide, South Australia, who first kindled my interest by asking me to teach classes in her private practice; Dr. Harry Rees, Medical Director, and staff of Physiotherapy Department of King Edward Memorial Hospital for Women, Perth, Western Australia, for unlimited freedom in trying new ideas; Margaret Farrant of the Department of Child Health, Perth, who initiated our joint teaching program at Bentley Hospital; and the support of many Perth obstetricians and gynecologists, particularly Drs. Colin Douglas-Smith, Andrew Kingsbury, and Archie Murray, whose concern for the nonsurgical treatment of pelvic floor problems initiated my interest in this field. I also wish to acknowledge the encouragement of Marjorie Ionta, Director of Physical Therapy at the Massachusetts General Hospital and Special Instructor in Physical Therapy at Simmons College, and the opportunity she provided me to teach childbirth education to undergraduate students in Boston. Pat Henderson, A.S.P.O.–certified Coordinator of the Maternity Teaching Program at Malden Hospital and my enthusiastic fellow teacher, is thanked for first introducing me to the childbirth scene in the Boston area and for her continuous assistance and support.

The following people were kind enough to read the manuscript and offer their valuable criticisms: Hans Kraus, M.D., Associate Professor of Physical Medicine and Rehabilitation, New York University; Llona Higgins, M.D., Tufts Medical School; Susie Hilbers, L.P.T., national teacher trainer for A.S.P.O.; Jim Little, L.P.T., certified Bradley teacher; Beth Shearer Conner of C/SEC; Pat Henderson, R.N.; Dr. Colin Douglas-Smith, F. R. C. O. G., Senior Obstetrician and Gynecologist, King Edward Memorial Hospital for Women, Perth. I am also fortunate that my editor, Anita McClellan, is similarly committed to the philosophy of women helping themselves and I am indebted to her insights and assistance. My husband also deserves special thanks for his patience, encouragement, and inestimable contributions to the manuscript.

Preface to the Second Edition

Elizabeth Noble stands out dramatically as one of the few women who have significantly affected the health care of childbearing women during the past decade. She combines a learned perception of human physiology with a common-sense approach to improving body mechanics and good health in general. Her own healthy good looks are evidence that she practices what she preaches.

Both providers and consumers of maternity care have greatly benefited from *Essential Exercises for the Childbearing Year* since its publication in 1976. The first book to address the postoperative needs of the caesarean mother, today it remains the only exercise guide that simply and clearly explains how the muscles of the body function through pregnancy, birth, and postpartum. Explanations are provided so that the reader understands the reasons for performing or avoiding certain movements and positions during pregnancy, labor, birth, and postpartum.

Elizabeth Noble has advanced childbirth education in the United States far beyond that of any other country. Her lectures and workshops, as well as the immense success of *Essential Exercises* over the past five years, have resulted in childbirth educators and hospitals taking a broader look at their educational programs for childbearing couples. The influence of *Essential Exercises* on physical therapists and nurses specializing in obstetrics and gynecology has been as great as on expectant parents and their childbirth educators. This second, revised edition is even more constructive.

Significant to the Revised Edition is the new, detailed discussion of labor and delivery in which the interaction of the different muscle groups and body systems are carefully described. Elizabeth Noble explains the need for a mother to avoid controlled breathing during labor in order to avoid mental and physical exhaustion. She also describes the need to avoid unnatural positions during labor and birth, which tend to inhibit the normal progress of childbirth.

Her explanation of how walking, standing, and sitting reduce the mother's discomfort and facilitate the progress of labor is particularly helpful. Medical research now supports this concept of ambulation during labor.

The adverse effects of prolonged breath-holding on the heart, lungs, and circulation of both mother and fetus, described in the book, have also been demonstrated since the book's original publication. Indeed, it was Elizabeth Noble's focus on this aspect of the birth process that instigated the corroborative research carried out by the renowned perinatologist Roberto Caldeyro-Barcia, M.D., immediate past president of the International Federation of Obstetricians and Gynecologists.

Throughout *Essential Exercises* the author stresses the importance of developing relaxation and awareness skills. Used together with normal breathing, they can help avoid tension, undue effort, and subsequent fatigue or exhaustion during labor. The chapter on relaxation has been revised to make clear that the more a childbearing woman can become in tune with her body during pregnancy the better she can repond to its natural rhythms during birth.

Elizabeth Noble founded the Obstetrics and Gynecology Section of the American Physical Therapy Association, and many physical therapists are now offering preventive and therapeutic exercise in this field. She is also a consultant, and recently participated in a film based on this book. It is to Elizabeth Noble's deserved credit that *Essential Exercises* has frequently been adopted as a text and resource for nursing and physical therapy obstetric programs as well as for childbirth education classes.

Doris Haire, D.M.S.
President, American Foundation for Maternal and Child Health, Inc.

Foreword

Obstetrics has yet to reap the full benefits of the discipline of physical therapy. Intuitively, one should expect these two fields of medicine to integrate naturally. It is difficult to understand, therefore, why there has been such reluctance — even overt negativism — to apply the well-grounded principles of physical therapy to fill the obvious needs of the obstetrical patient. To illustrate, the late W. C. W. Nixon denigrated exercise programs roundly as "just a peg on which to hang instructions." His attitude was all the more remarkable because he served as director of the natural childbirth program at the University College Hospital in London.

Adoption and acceptance of the principles of physical therapy as applied to childbirth preparation has been spotty at best even though it was formally introduced and pursued more than three decades ago by such staunch advocates as Helen Heardman. Popularization of a wide variety of exercise programs as components of psychoprophylactic regimens attests to the newer and growing awareness on the part of women in our culture and their collective demand for active participation. This has brought about a gratifying reexamination of all aspects of the rituals of the labor and delivery process. Although this trend has not necessarily been warmly received by obstetrical attendants everywhere, physicians have increasingly assessed their procedures. Within limits of safety, some are being discarded, including items once considered routine and essential, such as predelivery shaving and enema. Heavy sedation is fortunately decried today. More natural means are being stressed for their proven benefits.

Latest to be reconsidered is the entire spectrum of physical therapy as it applies not only to the delivery process, but as preparation for pregnancy and the postpartum recovery period. This is not a new idea, by any means. It is difficult to conceive why it has taken so many decades to be "rediscovered." In the United States, we are far behind our colleagues abroad, but even they have not fully embraced all relevant concepts (with the possible exception of the "mother gymnasts" of Scandinavia). When exercise is used as part of childbirth preparation, it is generally concentrated exclusively on aspects related to labor and delivery.

What is of great interest, of course, is that there is little uniformity or consistency to their (or our) recommendations and objectives. There is almost a capricious arbitrariness about the exercise programs of the several prevailing "schools." It is as if the birth process were somehow different among women in different geographical areas. Each group has its adherents and each claims to be effective and useful.

It is little wonder that deprecatory remarks are generated about exercise by knowledgeable people. Yet all have the same roots — in theory at least — and the same aims insofar as the pregnant woman is concerned. C. L. Buxton (*A Study of Psychophysical Methods for Relief of Childbirth Pain*, W. B. Saunders Company, Philadelphia, 1962) openly questioned the diversity of exercise programs by showing that "exercises carried out . . . to fit local philosophies and needs seem to be somewhat aimless." He seriously doubted the value of ". . . [a] purposeless exercise program persisted in because it was conventional to do so."

Why such wide discrepancies? The answer must surely lie in the lack of substantive support for any one of the programs in terms of scientific proof. This is not meant to imply that they are not useful and worthy, but merely to point out that none has been shown to be particularly better than any other, nor has there been any attempt made to optimize the benefits of such programs by improving them progressively by periodic objective evaluations of various modifications. Without such critical periodic evaluations, it is too easy for the casual observer or participant to be deluded by testimonials to good results. Anecdotal support is helpful, to be sure, but it is far from infallible and does not provide the kind of unbiased objectivity we especially need when we are dealing with matters of a subjective nature that appear to generate strong emotions by protagonists and antagonists alike.

The aims of this book are summarized in the single sentence "The childbearing year is both a season and a goal for which physical preparation and restoration is essential and rewarding." The concept of the year of pregnancy and recovery interval includes the critical postpartum period and involves the often-neglected rehabilitative aspects necessitating rapid return of physical efficiency and stamina. Without the kind of physical (and mental) preparation that the pregnant woman should experience, the labor and delivery process is less effective or well tolerated, and subsequent recovery may be retarded. The key here is prevention and the author offers a minimal but effective program toward this end.

The material is presented in a straightforward, no-nonsense and practical manner. It is neither condescending nor patronizing; it is mature and literate and is authoritative without being dogmatic. It provides clear-cut rationale where logical justifications are available. The discussions are sensible and realistic, although there are some contentious and arguable points raised that may not be entirely acceptable to obstetricians at large (for example, categorically assailing episiotomy). But the hyperbole should not detract from the primary thrust of the book or from its important and meaningful objectives.

There is a natural and edifying sequence of information concerning basic principles, functions of muscle groups, the changes that occur during pregnancy, labor, and postpartum, the kinds of problems one may encounter, details of exercise programs, and valuable hints on misconceptions, errors, shortcomings, and prohibitions. Needless to say, the pregnant woman would be well advised to check out specifics with her doctor, particularly before embarking on the recommended exercise programs; but within any constraints that he or she may impose, the rewards will be great.

The impact of physical therapy has long been recognized and applauded in other "rehabilitative" situations ranging from orthopedic problems and stroke to postmastectomy. Its potential in obstetrics is still to be realized. We are pleased in the Obstetrical Unit at the Beth Israel Hospital in Boston to be involved with Elizabeth Noble in propagating the concepts and practices expounded here by her. We expect her efforts will serve to stimulate a revival of interest in this important field for the real benefits it will bring to pregnant women everywhere.

Emanuel A. Friedman, M.D., Med.Sc.D.
Professor of Obstetrics and Gynecology
Harvard Medical School
Obstetrician-Gynecologist-in-Chief
Beth Israel Hospital
Boston, Massachusetts

1 Pregnancy Creates a Special Need for Exercise

FOR MANY DECADES, various techniques have been available to assist a woman in preparing for the exciting event of birth. The popularity of training for childbirth continues to increase as women, and couples, decide to participate as fully as they can in an experience that, in these days, may occur only once or twice in a lifetime.

Often the commitment to prepare for the drama of labor and delivery obscures the needs of the body while it undergoes vast adaptation during the childbearing year — from conception through postpartum adjustment. Physical preparation is important during pregnancy, and even more important is the need for restoration afterward, a fact that is frequently overlooked by American women and their doctors. Whether an expectant mother plans a hospital or home birth, with or without anesthesia, her muscles, joints, and tissues undergo changes and are subject to stress. If she is to be at her best throughout these months and if she is to prevent future problems, it is essential that she improve her physical condition to meet these burdens. This need applies to all childbearing women whether they are having their first or fifth baby.

In a way, the process is like giving a party. One always forgets how much work is necessary during the period of planning and anticipation. The actual event seems to pass quickly because we are excited and preoccupied. After the party is over, there's a lot more work to be done before the house gets back into shape and working order again. Similarly, the body undergoes hormonal and physical changes, which occur gradually during the long months of pregnancy, but after delivery these changes are reversed within a matter of weeks. Labor and delivery thus signify both an end and a beginning. The lengthy period of waiting and preparation is over, and so is the hard physical effort and excitement of the actual birth. But the greatest change and stress of the childbearing year occur after the arrival of the baby. Your physical, emotional, and psychological needs are more pronounced then than they are in pregnancy, yet it is at this time that your rehabilitation may be neglected because of your preoccupation with the newborn and its demands. The rapid return of your physical efficiency and stamina is very necessary, especially if you are planning to resume work soon, or will be caring for additional children at home.

Birth is a natural physiological event, but this creative process may be accompanied by potential destructive factors that place your body at risk. Just as you would equip your car with snow tires if you expected it to weather heavy winter conditions, so you must see to it that the body has the extra help it needs in its physical development, to provide support for the growing baby without causing the mother undue strain or gynecological problems. The inevitable changes that occur during pregnancy include the stretching of muscles, softening of ligaments, and loosening of joints in order to make more room inside. But whether the external and internal structural supports of the body are adequate to meet and recover from these changes is far from inevitable — it depends on you. The muscles supporting the backbone, and those in front of and beneath the pelvis, are put under great stress, which alters their function if care is not taken. You must exercise and maintain the voluntary muscles over which you do have control. Such exercise will provide significant benefits not only throughout the maternity cycle but for the rest of your life as well. During the birth, however, additional expenditure of voluntary muscles is often not needed — the uterus works by itself to ensure that the baby is born with or without your contribution. Training for this event, then, is more for coordination and relaxation than for maternal physical exertion. After delivery the uterus continues its involuntary contractions, and within six weeks it will return to its original state. But only your physical efforts will return the other muscles to their former size and function.

From childhood on, we've been told we should exercise more, along with reminders to sit up straight, and not to stand round-shouldered. Unfortunately for most people, the real value of exercise has not been well promoted in the past and opportunities may have been limited. At school, for example, competition was usually emphasized at the expense of enjoyment, body-building at the expense of flexibility exercises or relaxation, the talented performers at the expense of the average person, and men at the expense of women. Today physical fitness for its own sake is becoming popular and its importance in preventing diseases associated with inactivity (obesity, heart ailments, emotional problems) is now acknowledged. Increasing numbers of people are making an effort to pursue regular exercise whether for duty or pleasure. One sees more women among neighborhood joggers, and the women's movement has helped the spread of group activities and classes in YWCAs and other centers. Despite this consciousness-raising, most of us still undertake merely seasonal fits of activity — if we do any at all — such as tackling the winter flab before venturing out in beach clothes or limbering up as the ski season approaches. Although we know that we would benefit from daily physical exercise, we are more likely to take the body for granted and to worry about making special efforts only when it seems threatened in some way or when we have in mind a goal that requires physical preparation.

The childbearing year is both a season and a goal for which physical preparation and restoration are essential and rewarding. Often the special needs of pregnancy are recognized only when they have not been attended to. The young mother may look aghast at her "ruined figure" after childbirth. Her self-esteem feels as collapsed as the sagging breasts, folds of flesh, and fallen arches. Some women, on the other hand, accept their "lot" with resignation and the typical excuse of "that's what having a baby does to you." These external signs are well-known, but the frequent internal disturbances may be less understood. Even if a woman is not concerned with appearances, she cannot welcome impairment of her body's function. A floppy belly is one thing, but problems with pelvic organ support, urine control, or comfort in intercourse are often as unnecessary as they are common. These symptoms, arising in connection with childbirth, may be slow to develop and may subtly manifest themselves as fatigue, frustration, and unhappiness. The signs may be ignored initially, but with the passage of years, and perhaps subsequent pregnancies, surgical repair may be necessary.

This book emphasizes the need for women to understand and control their bodies. The key concept is prevention. Gaining knowledge and foresight in order to prevent unnecessary problems is the best approach to health care. Since the childbearing year is not a time of illness, grasping and executing some of the essentials must be seen as an education, not a treatment. It is simply a woman's responsibility to herself during a natural, although burdensome, process. While this process may be inevitable, your response or lack of it is not. You

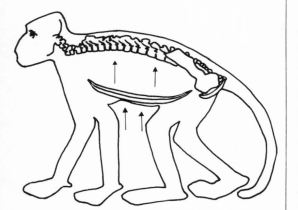

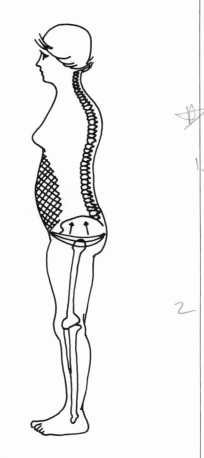

The abdominal and pelvic floor muscles reversed roles when humans became upright.

can establish a lasting pattern in which exercise maintains optimum muscle strength and length, relieves nervous tension, enhances the benefits of good nutrition, and thus becomes an essential component of healthy living. The course of human evolution, and the development of some cultural habits that encourage physical softness, can help explain why women today need, more than ever before, to exercise prior to and during pregnancy and postpartum.

Pregnancy accentuates some of the potential problems inherent in human evolutionary development. Unlike the brain and the hand, which have undergone amazing refinement, the grosser, more basic parts of the body have progressed little in evolutionary terms. When humans stood on two legs, the structural supporting system became modified and the role of muscles in supporting the bony framework and its contents in the upright position became paramount. But our urban way of life, which allows the underexercise of most muscles and the persistent stress on others, has caused certain parts of the body to merge as points of structural weakness and potential trouble spots. These are most significantly, the backbone, the abdominal muscles, and the layers of muscles forming the floor to the pelvic cavity.

The backbone had to develop curves to counteract the forces of compression that gravity causes in the erect posture. During pregnancy these curves become more pronounced as the body's weight enlarges and its center of gravity moves forward in relation to the spine. If adequate muscular support is lacking, this increase in stress causes the pelvis to tip forward and posture to be poor, which commonly results in fatigue and backache since the back muscles are forced to do work for which they were not designed. The more s-shaped the spinal column, the more these muscles are taxed.

The abdominal muscles, which support the spine against gravity in four-legged animals, do very little in the vertical position that humans customarily assume. They do even less work in our industrialized society because we mostly sit or stand. These muscles, during pregnancy, have the task of supporting the growing weight of the baby and are consequently required to be stronger and more elastic than they usually are. As a tomato plant, when laden with fruit, tends to droop forward and needs to be splinted to a support, so the abdominal muscles become stretched over the pregnant uterus and, if further weakened through neglect or incorrect use, will strain rather than support the backbone.

3 The pelvic floor,* in contrast with the abdominal muscles, has had to do much more work since humans became upright. It must withstand the forces of gravity and increased pressure within the body (such as is incurred during straining, lifting, elimination), and must also support the pelvic organs. For all this, we humans have just a sling of muscle at the base of our trunks. In four-legged animals the muscles are much more extensive, arising from the whole of the pelvic brim. While we don't have a tail to wag, we do have the power to move the pelvic floor muscles to counteract the effects to which they are subjected. However, this necessary muscle action is poorly developed in most women. Pregnancy further jeopardizes the vulnerable pelvic floor because of the increased weight it must support as the uterus enlarges. During delivery the baby passes through the pelvic floor by way of the vagina, which means that the whole supportive sheet is greatly stretched and may, indeed, be injured.

Our forebears had to contend with these potential problems in human architecture and babies have always come out the same way, of course, so what has changed? Our physical condition. With the march of modern civilization we have become more and more removed from the routine physical work that compensates for these structural weaknesses by muscular development. Women in our society rely on armchairs, automobiles, and on various kinds of labor-saving devices to free them for leisure activities. But these activities, too, may exclude physical exertion. Obviously our muscles are underutilized when compared with those of women who, say, work in fields or perform domestic functions, such as washing, preparing and cooking food while squatting, or sitting without the support of a chair. If you've ever dined on the floor of a traditional Japanese restaurant, you'll know how accustomed your body has become to furniture! Our cultural and personal habits have as much effect or more on the physical state of our bodies as do evolutionary or other inherited factors.

The best way to meet the physical challenges of the childbearing experience is to understand their nature and to act. Do not wait until you are forced to react, for this may mean joining the crowded waiting rooms of orthopedic or gynecological specialists. Recuperation then can be a real problem for a woman,

---

* Also known as the perineum, perineal area, levator ani, pubo-coccygeus, Kegel muscle, pelvic or urogenital diaphragm.

since so many of her household duties are often still unavoidable and will aggravate the conditions, especially fatigue
and backache.

Preparation for childbirth and restoration afterward is not
complicated or strenuous. Dancing or athletic skills are neither
required nor developed, as some books on prenatal and postpartum exercises seem to imply! Actually, you need to do many
more of the easier exercises and far fewer of the harder ones.
Moreover, you need to know the rationale for the exercise that
you are doing or not doing. It's like selecting the most nutri-
tious items in the supermarket when many other items of
dubious value may look or taste good. A decision-making process is involved, and in order to make an informed choice you
need to know certain facts. Since there are plenty of publications that offer a general keep-fit regime, this manual will focus
on the essential aspects of female physique during the childbearing year. The aim is to provide a minimal, effective program for the woman with little time or little inclination to exercise, or the woman who has doubts about what is wise and
safe in her condition — and for all women, whether they would
exercise at any other time or not, who realize that special needs
must be met in pregnancy and postpartum.

The actual exercises are described following detailed evaluations of the needs of the body at the various stages of the
childbearing year. By focusing on significant parts of the body
and their changing role, you will, it is hoped, be motivated to
ease the adjustments and give yourself the best preventive care.
If you learn to recognize early signs of weakness and dysfunction, you can usually reverse these problems with corrective
exercise. The key muscles involved in childbearing are just not
adequately exercised during housework, neighborhood strolls,
or playing an occasional sport. Significantly, pregnancy
worsens the potential structural weaknesses of the muscles
modified when human beings became upright creatures. You
will notice in the exercise schemes that it is these very muscles
that you prepare before birth and the same ones that you re-.
store afterward.

No program is complete unless it includes ways to achieve
relaxation and good breathing habits. Their importance in the
sequence of pregnancy, labor, delivery, and postpartum will be
discussed as well. Your mate, other family members, and even
friends can benefit from practicing these techniques, which will
be of lasting value for the rest of your life.

Prenatal Exercises

One goal of prenatal exercises is to adjust the body so that it can better carry the load of pregnancy, and in the most general sense this means developing good posture. You learn how to align the parts of your body, in whatever position you assume (particularly one's habitual posture in standing and in working), so that joints are protected from strain and you don't waste energy with unnecessary muscle use. Exercises to achieve these aims will also help prevent much of the discomfort, postural backache, and fatigue that plague most women — pregnant or not — since they spend so much time leaning over counters and sinks, peering into ovens or fridges, and reaching down to children and objects on the floor.

Postural problems are common in pregnancy because the body has to adapt to structural changes, which alter its center of gravity, and to hormonal changes, which affect the stability of joints. Consequently, the alignment and balance of the body segments must adjust with these changes. These adjustments occur mostly at a subconscious level because of automatic righting reflexes. Together they form a complex mechanism that enables the body to know its position in space, so we can get around without looking at our feet, holding on to things, or falling over. However, if poor postural habits have been developed over the years, they will need evaluation and correction. During pregnancy women tend to stand farther back on their heels because the center of gravity moves forward as the weight increases in front. Some compensate for this backward shift, perhaps, by tilting the pelvis farther forward, hollowing more at the base of the spine, or swaying back from the waist. Whatever the form, it is uncomfortable and unattractive.

Most of us don't realize our posture is faulty until we experience some symptoms of pain or deformity. These may not arise for many years, by which time muscles and other tissues will have shortened or stretched. But in pregnancy, symptoms resulting from poor posture appear much more quickly, whether from a latent weakness or a disturbance of postural reflexes as well as the normal hormonal softening of ligaments. As the center of gravity moves forward, activity in the back muscles is increased. The muscles may become so stretched or weakened in front, or tensed and shortened in the back, that they do not respond to the stretch stimulus that normally helps maintain good posture at a reflex level. So the bones and ligaments become overloaded because the muscles are not doing their share.

The childbearing state does not mean that a woman must suffer poor posture. On the contrary, exercise and re-education have great value. Re-education means that the stronger muscle fibers help the weaker ones along until the whole muscle is working together again. Obviously, unlearning bad habits, which may have existed for a long time, requires more effort than simply learning and keeping good ones. The general aim of exercises and postural training is to enable you not only to see the difference but to feel it. When this is achieved at a conscious level, then it must be adequately reinforced to cause a transfer to subconscious levels of control. This way you can offer your body the best protection against a sudden back lesion occurring from a minor trauma. Research done by Professor Hans Kraus of New York University showed that 80 percent of cases of back pain are due to lack of adequate physical activity. Only a very small percentage of lower back pain is of gyneco-logical origin. A discussion of positions and body mechanics is included to help you avoid strain or injury and poor working habits. The joints of the body become loosened under the influence of the increased hormone production during preg-nancy which softens ligaments and fibrous tissue. The muscles of the lower abdomen and buttocks, if kept strong, can help protect their associated pelvic joints. Learning to substitute squatting to floor level rather than leaning from your waist is an example of how you can maintain mobility of the joints, but at the same time protect them by a stable position of minimal strain.

Exercises for the abdominal muscles maintain the muscles' elastic qualities so that they can better support the pelvis and its contents, including the growing baby. Gas and constipation are more frequent when there is sluggish intestinal activity result-ing from a slack abdominal wall and insufficient exercise. The muscles need to be as elastic as possible, since they undergo great stretching to accommodate the baby and may even be strained apart toward the end of pregnancy or during labor. Weakness or separation reduces the ability of the abdominal muscles to assist in the expulsion of the baby down the birth canal in the second stage of labor. Backache can occur in a first pregnancy or later ones, because the back muscles are forced to compensate for the abdominals in holding the spine erect.

The goal of pelvic floor exercises, too, is to keep the mus-

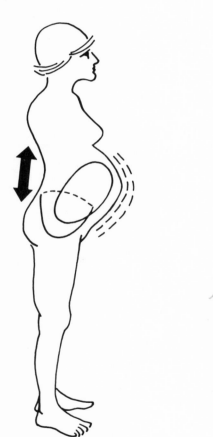

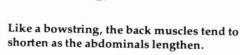

Like a bowstring, the back muscles tend to shorten as the abdominals lengthen.

cles strong and supportive when there is added stress from the enlarging uterus, which the softening pelvic floor must uphold. Another important benefit of these exercises is that a supple, healthy muscle will allow more distention of the vagina during delivery. Consistent use of these muscles can also alleviate the problems of constipation and poor blood circulation (such as varicose veins of the pelvic area, the most common form of which is hemorrhoids) as well as improve your sex life. Learning to contract the pelvic floor muscles is necessary if one is to prevent undue sagging, with downward displacement of pelvic organs, at any time of your life. The power in these muscles is most often entirely neglected, which is ironical when their fundamental role in female health and happiness is considered. Another good reason for prenatal exercise of the pelvic floor is that your task of restoration will be much easier if you know how to tighten the muscles before they are stretched during birth. This prenatal standard will be your guide; you will not have to try to learn the action for the first time when the muscles are slack.

Training for relaxation provides you with a skill that will be valuable for the rest of your life, not only during pregnancy and labor. Relaxation is more than just rest. You learn to release tension — and muscles can be tense and tight as well as weak. Since we express emotions as well as carry out movement and actions with our muscles, even the most subtle mental irritation can influence the state of our muscles. In the hassles of daily living, most of our anger and annoyance is suppressed; this accumulates stress in the body systems. Regular relaxation helps things to go much more smoothly during the childbearing year and later, when you have to cope with even more noises, interruptions, and anxious moments. Exercises and relaxation obviously are most essential on those frustrating days when you feel the most pressed and are likely to skip them.

Good breathing habits need to be developed, especially when exercising, since both mother and baby benefit from an optimum supply of oxygen during pregnancy and labor. Slow, deep breathing aids the blood circulation and its soothing rhythm helps the mother to relax. Breathing patterns requiring mental concentration are commonly taught as distraction techniques during labor contractions. For some women this is a way of coping with discomfort. However, any control of an involuntary process, such as breathing, interferes with relaxation. Most of us quicken our respiration under stress but over-breathing (hyperventilation) during contractions must be prevented. Excessive breathing results in an oxygen surplus for the mother (if carried to extremes this will cause her to faint) and has the *reverse* effect of a decreased oxygen supply for the baby. Easy, relaxed breathing maintains the best physiological balance, keeps you in a psychological state of calm, and confidence, and conserves your energy.

Walking, swimming, and bicycling are enjoyable activities that not only provide excellent general exercise but bring you into the fresh air and sunshine. Done regularly, they combine many of the desirable features of prenatal exercise planning: to strengthen muscles, build up endurance, improve circulation and respiration, adapt to increasing weight and changing balance. They are pleasant diversions, available to almost everyone, and help to burn up extra calories if you are overweight and to relieve constipation. These activities, now commonly referred to as aerobics, emphasize the improvement of heart and lung performance — reaching a certain peak within a given time period. This promotes better overall function of the body and increases its ability to accommodate exertion. Aerobic exercise differs from calisthenics which focus on developing strength, flexibility, and coordination of muscles, and improving joint mobility. One should be concerned with both approaches for complete conditioning. While some relaxation of the pelvic joints is normal in pregnancy, the degree of joint instability and any associated discomfort varies. Many women maintain a jogging program right through the ninth month and resume it a few weeks postpartum but some expectant mothers experience difficulty and pain when walking in late pregnancy. In rare cases, this results from a considerable separation at the union of the pubic bones and activities which involve hip motion should be limited. (These sensations occur specifically in the central pubic area and must be distinguished from the commonly-felt pressure and discomfort in the groin.)

While prenatal exercises build the body and provide other benefits so that the burdens of pregnancy may be met more efficiently and comfortably, they do not shorten your labor to an appreciable degree. Of course, your being in good physical condition can enhance the contribution you make through greater relaxation and cooperation in the first stage (where your role is passive and the uterus works by itself) and effective bearing-down in the second stage (when you work actively to assist the uterus in pushing the baby down the birth canal). If you are physically fit you cope better with both mental and physical stress. You will have greater endurance if your labor is long or arduous. Your confidence is increased when you know that your body is strong and healthy; by the same token poor physical condition and being overweight decrease the feeling of well-being.

Preparation classes for the event of childbirth are strongly recommended. Supervision and group interaction are acknowledged to be positive factors in any educational undertaking. Discussing experiences with other expectant parents makes you feel less isolated, and there is always something to be learned from others. A partner-coach who trains with you is of great value in sharing your emotional growth at this time, boosting your morale, and providing reassurance as well as assistance with comfort and physical techniques for labor. The educated expectant mother, with or without a support-person, is able to cooperate with her body and the people assisting her for whatever the type of labor and the delivery it may be her luck to experience. Understanding the process of labor is very important so that the couple gains trust and confidence in the body's ability to perform its natural functions. They also need to know their rights and responsibilities with regard to the increasing medical interference in childbirth. Studies have shown that preparation and participation in the birth process reduce the need for medication and obstetrical intervention. The actual birth takes less than a day; the nature of events is outside the mother's control. Preparation for this occasion may be intense and extensive. This is justifiable and essential because birth is the exciting climax. In contrast, the states of pregnancy and postpartum, with their immense changes, endure for months, and the physical outcome of their management may also have far-reaching effects. It seems logical, then, to view training for these adaptive phases as equally important. Significantly, the muscles that require preparation and restoration, unlike the uterus, are under voluntary control.

When to Start Prenatal Exercises

Exercises can be begun at any time and continued through life since they pertain to optimum function of the female body. Women who seek advice or instruction regarding prenatal exercises usually do so in the last trimester. The basic exercise scheme is designed for these women, who are six months pregnant or more. Fortunately, movement and fitness classes for early pregnancy are becoming more available. Women should begin exercising as soon as possible, even before they conceive. Then they can undertake a progressive exercise plan in addition, modifying the exercises in later pregnancy as they feel necessary. The greatest value of exercise, however, is during the recovery period. So if you have established a regular program before the baby arrives, it will be much easier to continue than it would be if you waited until afterward, especially in light of the added distractions you will have then. It will be easier on you mentally, because you have already made the commitment to prepare and restore your body. And it will be easier physically, because a healthy, active muscle regains its shape, elasticity, and function much sooner than one that has been neglected. Don't despair if you are reading this in the maternity ward of the hospital: it is never too late. On the contrary, this work is even more important for you.

Postpartum Exercises

At this time you will concentrate on restoring the body as quickly as you can to its state of efficiency that existed before pregnancy. The idea that, since the body took nine months to complete the pregnancy, another nine are required to reverse all the effects is quite wrong. Physiological changes occur in hours and days, and exercises show results in days and weeks.

Postural habits need to be re-established so that you don't continue the stance you had in pregnancy. This means you must consciously contract the abdominal and pelvic floor muscles at first, in order to balance the pelvis again after the sudden loss of its load.

Because of the hormonal effects of pregnancy, the joints remain at risk for some weeks, and good body mechanics are even more essential at this time to protect them and their ligaments until the muscles regain their former length and strength.

The abdominal muscles after delivery display the most obvious need for attention. The goal of postpartum exercises is to restore them to their original state. Exercises are designed to shorten and eventually strengthen them, so that you achieve a flat abdomen and good posture with the pelvis tilted back to realign in its correct relationship to the spine. Before you attempt stronger exercises, a self-check, described in Chapter 3, must be made to see if any separation of the muscles in the midline has occurred.

The purpose of pelvic floor exercises after delivery is to tighten the muscles to enable them to resume their role in supporting the pelvic contents, and to re-establish sphincter control. After birth the muscles will feel very slack and stretched, and it is imperative that they not be allowed to remain in this state. The longer you postpone their restoration, the more muscle atrophy and tissue degeneration will take place. Because the pelvic floor muscles are not easily or completely observed, your most reliable guide is how they function. Their weakness has far greater ramifications for a woman than does weakness of the abdominal muscles, although laxity of the abdominal wall is more conspicuous. It is important that you fully comprehend the function of the pelvic floor and any indicators of trouble. With this knowledge you will be in a position to evaluate the results of your restorative work and to assess the state of the muscles before progressing with abdominal exercises. This is an important point, because strong abdominal work causes increased pressure on the pelvic floor, which can strain and further weaken the muscles if their withstanding power is inadequate. Breathing is coordinated, with exhaling on exertion.

After delivery you will need much rest and sleep, and relaxation is very important at this time. Lying on your front with a pillow under the hips is a good way to achieve this, and it is a particularly comfortable position for encouraging the pelvic organs to resume their normal places.

Postpartum exercises are easier to perform if you have practiced them beforehand. Your muscles are prepared — and so are you. But in any case, they should never be omitted. They are necessary if the body is to be restored to its former condition, and they provide increasing protection during this altered and vulnerable state of the body. Nature takes care of internal changes, such as the shrinkage of the uterus, but only you can bring about a change in the slackness of the voluntary muscles.

The following chapters will enable you to supervise your own postpartum program. Exercises should be modified to allow for the different body and different birth experience of each individual. The return in muscle strength varies from woman to woman, and from muscle to muscle in the same person. It makes no sense, then, to pick up a booklet that states, "On Day 3, repeat Exercise B 10 times." Arbitrary instructions, furthermore, make no allowances for any defect in the abdominal wall or pelvic floor, nor is the interaction between the abdominal muscles and pelvic floor considered, which can mean that one group of muscles gets strong at the expense of the other. People rarely fit into rigidly defined categories, especially during the childbearing year. I have tried to supply as much information as possible to help women understand their bodies. This way they can avoid exercises that are pointless or harmful, such as double-leg–raising, soon after birth, because they will recognize that muscle length and tone must be restored before the muscles can be expected to perform strongly. Signs and symptoms of strain and weakness are described so that women can evaluate their own abdominal and pelvic floor muscles. With this knowledge they can progress or modify the exercises according to their own body feedback instead of blindly following some conventional program.

When to Start Postpartum Exercises

Exercises after delivery should be begun as soon as possible — certainly within 24 hours. Muscle work involved in immediate postpartum exercises is not strenuous or in any way potentially harmful. Patients who have had major surgery — a much greater ordeal than childbirth — do such exercises the first day, so it is unlikely that you would be unable to do them for any medical reason. The exercises must be done for short periods and often — not in long, tiring sessions. The muscles have been stretched: these exercises will coax them back into shape and encourage their return to their former length and tone. This initial step must be achieved before any strengthening programs involving resistive exercises are embarked upon.

Don't entertain the idea that you'll take it easy for the first week or so, and at some later date start on a crash program of fancy physical jerks. The greatest changes occur in the first week or so. Furthermore, you need to be in reasonable shape before resuming household tasks, being an active parent, and so on, or your fatigue, aches, and discomforts will multiply. Deficient muscles make you vulnerable to sudden development of back pain from even a very minor cause. If you deliver in the hospital, this is the best place to begin exercises. Do not wait until you get home, where the new routine (or lack of it) will make it very difficult for you to find the time and inclination to get started. You have the greatest need for them during these early days as well as the best opportunity to do them. This is very important. You will be amazed at what you can achieve during your brief hospital stay.

When you stop to think about it, hardly anything we do

comes naturally; it is learned from others. Childbearing is a fundamental biological process, but since it is also a social and cultural process, it has given rise to fear, ignorance, superstition, and myths. These influences should have no place in modern society, where opportunities for information and education now exist and advances in medical technology have made childbirth safer than crossing the road. However, the increasing medicalization of birth causes many couples to feel that the process is no longer natural. Emotional and psychological preparation are just as important as physical preparation; women should feel secure and self-reliant, and trust in their own bodies and resources. The responsibility of women today is to become informed consumers, especially when they become mothers.

Women, by the very nature of their reproductive system, will always be more involved than men in the use and abuse of health care. And it will take some time to reverse the ironical situation in which men are usually the providers of health care in our society. If women can understand and evaluate their own physical needs with a view to prevention, the less they'll need to rely on others to provide a cure. In the case of exercise during the childbearing year, judgments are required that essentially involve personal body awareness and feedback. Besides — how often is any muscle testing included in a medical check-up? Women themselves must become qualified to make these subjective judgments, and to do so on the basis of objective physiological facts.

In sum, the formula for the best possible total birth experience must be conscious participation throughout the complete sequence — pregnancy, labor, delivery, and postpartum. You are not the director in the drama of your birth — the uterus calls the cues. Of course you must be awake and aware to play your part. Assisting nature to provide the best physical props and the tidiest dismantling afterward is also your responsibility. Keeping your body in top form during pregnancy, and ensuring its successful restoration postpartum, is within your power — and your power alone.

General Tips for Exercising

1. Start off slowly; warm up your system. Build up to the more demanding exercises and taper off gradually. A good way to taper off is to work back through the exercises in reverse order.

2. Do not overdo the amount of exercise in the beginning. It is easy to do too much because your muscles don't protest until the day after!

3. Exercise a few times but often. Avoid tiring sessions. Rest and relaxation are very important, too. Try to incorporate exercises into your daily routine activities:

- Tighten the abdominal wall when standing or sitting.
- Contract the pelvic floor during intercourse.
- Get on all fours to pick up, wash floors, and so forth.
- Squat to lift any object — light or heavy.
- Sit on the floor like a tailor, (with knees out and ankles crossed) to watch TV.
- Rotate ankles while feet are elevated.
- Rotate shoulders after feeding baby.
- Check posture each time you pass a mirror.

4. If you feel breathless, dizzy, or tired, stop and rest. Take your time. During physical activity waste products build up, which can cause muscles to quiver or bring on general fatigue, until the body adapts. Before arising from the horizontal position, especially after relaxation, stretch the whole body a couple of times and take one or two deep breaths. If resting on your back, roll onto your side before sitting up.

5. Do not hold your breath during exercises. An exercise that causes you to hold your breath is too strenuous. This increase in pressure can strain the abdominal wall or the pelvic floor. Breathing can be coordinated with exercises, such as pulling in or contracting the abdominal muscles on OUTWARD breath. A helpful guide is to exhale as you exert during any physical activity.

6. Exercises should be performed slowly and completely. You should always be comfortable and in control of both the position and the exercise. Stretching and limbering activities must be done gently and never forced. Avoid activities like pushing, pulling, or leaning in such a way that balance can be lost and muscles strained.

The "bicycling exercise" such as opposite, favors only round shoulders and a head that pokes forward! This position and also the "candlestick" are difficult maneuvers during the

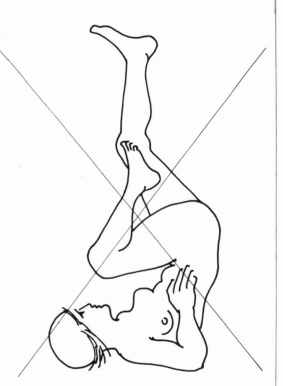

Bicycling

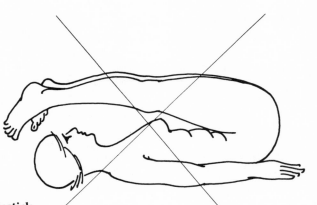

The Candlestick

childbearing year and they are potentially harmful as you could lose control at any point.

7. Avoid exercises that involve a lot of leverage. This simply means that the longer the lever — the greater amount of power required to move it. For example, much force (and strain) is generated when you try to raise both outstretched legs. Leverage is a principle by which exercises are progressed — not begun.

NEVER DO DOUBLE-LEG-RAISING as shown below, during the childbearing year, although it is often recommended. Indeed, the use of double-leg–raising as an exercise at any time to

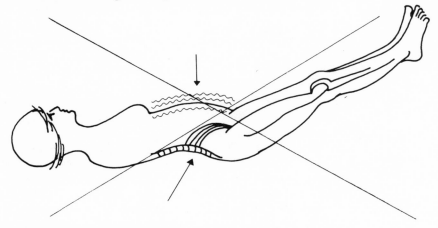

Raising both legs can strain the lower back.

strengthen the abdominal muscles is not justified by the anatomical facts. The abdominal muscles do not raise the legs. They work to stabilize the lower back — but at a great mechanical disadvantage when the length and weight (leverage) of the legs is considered. It is very difficult for the abdominal muscles to hold the back flat and so protect the vertebral joints against the stronger pull of the hip flexors which lift the legs and are attached to those joints. Invariably, the backbone arches under this strain, and if this happens repeatedly, orthopedic problems can develop. During pregnancy and postpartum, the stretched abdominal muscles are unable to stabilize the lower back as the legs are raised, so exercising in this way can actually impair the abdominal muscles and cause damage to the spinal joints.

8. Avoid positions and exercises that increase the hollow in the back. Excessive hollowing of the small of the back (lumbar region) is most undesirable, particularly if it is forced. This puts great stress on the already stretched abdominal muscles and compression on spinal joints. The ligaments, which have been softened in pregnancy, can be strained, leading to back pain. If the ligaments are persistently stretched during the postpartum recovery phase, the shortening that normally occurs at this time may be permanently impaired. Many of these positions are used in yoga and may be resumed after the childbearing year. Good yoga programs consist of a balance between all movements so that backward bending is complemented by forward bending. Supervision and absence of back pain are prerequisites for students beginning yoga.

9. Exercise in different places and positions. For variety, try a session with your partner, child, or a friend. The important thing is that the exercises are easy to do and can be done in many ways without requiring equipment or preparation. Most exercise programs are adamant about the use of the floor, since beds (although they should be very firm) are usually too soft for exercises requiring large movements with much effort. Certainly for the progressive abdominal exercises, the floor — with carpet, rug, blanket, or beachtowel — is most suitable. However, all the essential exercises in the summary sheets at the back of the book can be performed on your bed. Of course, this is the only practical place for postpartum exercises in the hospital. Warming-up in the morning, preparing for your afternoon rest and relaxation, or getting ready to sleep — you're on the

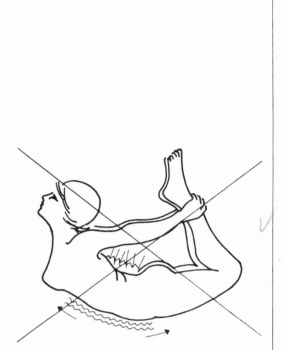

Exercises like this one strain the weakest points in the childbearing body.

bed and the opportunity is there. Toward the end of pregnancy, many women find it difficult to get up after lying down for a while on a very hard surface. As well as being uncomfortable lying on the back can cause low blood pressure when the increased weight of the uterus interferes with the circulation.

10. How many times should an exercise be performed? Since everyone is different, it makes no sense to advise a set number of repetitions. Alternation rather than repetition of the same muscle groups is always recommended when exercising. Multi-repetitions tend to cause fatigue and stiffness. Do just 4 to 5 and then change to another exercise. This is the basis of the schemes summarized on pages 163-169; exercises are interchanged as much as focus on the key groups permits. Pregnancy is a time to become more in tune with your body, so use the exercises for increasing your awareness of your breathing, muscles, joints, and posture. Muscles must be contracted AND relaxed, so it is important to rest briefly between exercises. Work within your own limit of comfort and tolerance. For example, stop before you are tired or if the muscles start to shake or if you do not have complete control of the movement. Breathing and heart rate should be normal before starting any exercise. You should not experience stiffness the next day. The benefits of exercise accrue with consistency and gentle progression. For prenatal exercises, progression occurs naturally with the advancing pregnancy, which provides increasing weight and resistance for the muscles to overcome, thus maintaining their strength and condition. Regular exercise is important to gain the best results and to avoid sudden strain. REMEMBER: Your rewards are what you yourself achieve!

The Pelvic Floor 2

IN ANY DISCUSSION of physical exercise during the childbearing year, the pelvic floor should receive top priority. These muscles have the greatest relevance to a woman's present and future condition, yet ironically they are the least well known. Women may have never heard or thought about the muscular power in this crucial center of their anatomy. Ideally, we should have learned its significance as children, or at least in school health or physical education classes. Exercises for the pelvic floor are left out of physical fitness books and may rate only a mention in a sex manual. The false impression is frequently given that the ability to use these muscles is either something you have or you don't have, on the checklist of what it takes to make a good sex partner. Even in childbirth education classes, the use of these muscles may be mentioned so briefly that students do not understand its importance. Postpartum re-education is almost certain to be neglected, although because of the immense trauma inflicted on the pelvic floor during birth this is the most essential area to exercise. Mothers reading this chapter will be able to train their daughters in pelvic floor exercises from early childhood.

Structure of the Pelvic Floor

The term *pelvic floor* conveys the idea of a base support (although it is not a rigid one but is suspended from bony points) and conveniently incorporates all the different muscles whose names and interaction complicate description. Try to visualize the position of these muscle layers, right between your legs, where they form the floor to the bony basin of the pelvis. This muscle sheet is also the base of support for the pelvic organs and their contents. The top of this abdominal-pelvic area is bounded by a broad muscle ceiling — the diaphragm — which separates it from the chest cavity.

The right and left halves of the pelvic floor unite in the midline, but the muscle sheet is penetrated by three orifices. Muscle fibers placed circularly around these openings form sphincters,

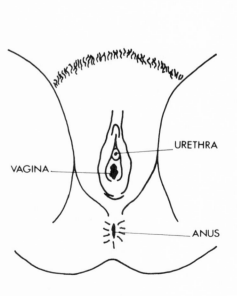

VAGINA

URETHRA

ANUS

Surface view of the perineum

interweaving also with the inner passages and the rest of the pelvic diaphragm. The strength of the muscular floor and the control of these sphincters are important in maintaining the integrity of the walls of the inside passages and the position of the organs they support.

The muscles form a figure 8 as they are slung in loops around the vaginal and urethral sphincter in front and the anal sphincter at the rear. The muscles and other tissue-supports are anchored in a firm fibrous node (the perineal body) between the anus and vagina. The significance of this is that the pelvic floor works as a coordinated whole, and the contraction of one sphincter in complete isolation from the other is not possible, although some claim to have accomplished this feat. The anal sphincter is the strongest and is usually held tightly closed except during elimination. What requires our attention is the front or "master" sphincter. Since the significant loop of muscle here is slung around both the vaginal and urethral openings, this means that the flow of urine is controlled by the same muscle action that occurs when the vagina is voluntarily constricted. This has important consequences for learning and checking the pelvic floor exercise, and will be discussed in detail later. This ring of muscle is also significant in sexual response, in order to achieve firm contact with the penis.

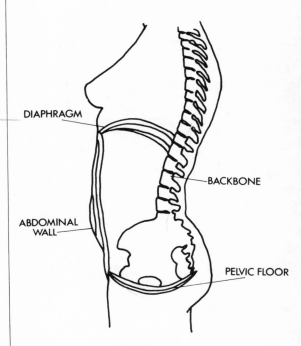

The boundaries of the pelvic cavity

Three openings penetrate the midline of the pelvic floor.

The muscles form a figure 8 around the perineal body.

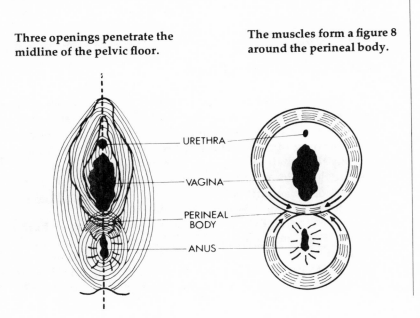

URETHRA

VAGINA

PERINEAL BODY

ANUS

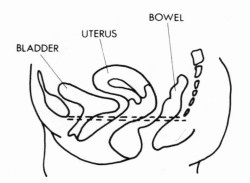

Good pelvic floor support with a firm base, organs in place

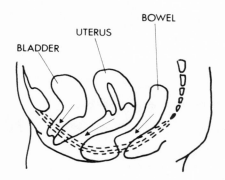

Inadequate support and the hammock sags, contents descend

The position of the pelvic floor, you recall, is at a greater disadvantage in humans due to the effects of gravity when we are in the upright position. Furthermore, the pelvic floor in humans although composed of several layers is just a hammock of muscle, suspended basically at two points, the front and the back of the pelvis, with minor attachments to the two bones that we sit on. The mechanics of this structural arrangement, plus gravity and the frequent increases of pressure within the body, make the pelvic floor likely to sag, just as a hammock does.

Ideally, the muscle floor is firm and supportive, forming a straight line between two bony points (pubis and coccyx). This is possible because it is composed of both voluntary and involuntary muscles, which are always in a state of partial contraction. The healthy, active pelvic floor, then, has tone and elasticity. (Tone in this sense meaning a normal firmness of tissues, which respond sufficiently to stretch and touch.) But when weakness or injury, commonly resulting from childbirth, causes the muscle floor to sag below the horizontal, it will continue its downward trend. What results is a very loose hammock, unless active attempts are made (through muscle re-education) to bring the pelvic floor back to its supportive role, maintaining the pelvic organs in their upright positions. Excessive sagging over a long period of time results in serious structural changes with consequent impairment of function.

Functions of the Pelvic Floor:

- To support the pelvic organs and their contents, most obviously the bladder, uterus, and bowel. Except under anesthesia, there is always some tone in the sphincters and surrounding muscles. These sphincters can be closed more tightly than their normal state of partial contraction and the pelvic floor drawn up into a more supportive position by the action of voluntary muscles, which are present in addition to the involuntary ones.
- To withstand all the increases in pressure that occur in the abdominal and pelvic cavity. The forces may be intermittent, such as those incurred by laughing, coughing, sneezing, lifting, straining, pushing during the second stage of labor, and elimination. Pregnancy, because of the

enlarging uterus, causes long-standing and increasing pressure on the pelvic floor.

- To provide sphincter control of the perineal openings. During elimination the pelvic floor relaxes and afterward contracts to return the muscles to their supportive state. Good sphincter control is an important factor in the basic strength of the floor. Voluntary control can be superimposed, as when we interrupt the stream of urine, or constrict the muscles in resistance to a vaginal or rectal examination or grip the penis during intercourse. It is also important that we be able voluntarily to relax the sphincters for pelvic examinations (and women experience plenty of these in their lifetime) and during delivery of the baby. The ability to release all the pelvic floor muscles as totally as possible is essential during the birth of the baby.

Since most women are not aware of either the functions or the importance of these muscles, it is unlikely that, at the outset, these are supple muscles over which you have good control. Your general fitness may be excellent, but this has no relation to the integrity of these internal structures. The pelvic floor is not exercised unintentionally during sports or calisthenics. Special efforts are required, although all that is involved is the act of uplifting the pelvic floor muscles and tightening the sphincters. The majority of women never bother to develop the power in these muscles and some may suffer no symptoms that indicate weakness of the pelvic floor. Why, then, should they concern themselves with exercises?

One worthwhile bonus is that your sex life may improve. The vagina becomes more snug as the muscles improve in strength and thickness. One can read in such books as the *Kamasutra* or *The Arabian Nights* of cultures where the ability to contract these muscles, namely, the vaginal sphincter, was encouraged and a highly prized asset. In some African tribes today, the young girls are not permitted to marry until they demonstrate good strength of the perineal muscles. They are similarly coached during postpartum by the discerning finger of the midwife.

A second reason for pelvic floor exercises is that problems can arise that are ultimately most distressing, though they may be slow to develop. These problems, which are exacerbated by childbirth, highlight the importance of proper pelvic floor function.

Common Problems with Pelvic Floor Function

The onset of these problems may be subtle; you may not experience a clear-cut symptom but the condition will worsen over the years if it goes unchecked. For example, you or your partner may feel nothing during intercourse, which could have to do with the laxity of the pelvic floor muscles. You may have difficulty retaining a tampon for the same reason. Sometimes the vaginal walls are so slack that other pelvic organs or the intestines protrude and cause discomfort. Most commonly, the problem is indicated by vague aches, fatigue, and dissatisfaction, and persists for a long time until the onset of symptoms that cause you to seek medical help. One such symptom is prolapse of the uterus, which progresses through several stages before it actually herniates through the vaginal outlet, similar to the way upholstery padding protrudes through a chair when its supporting base is defective.

Urinary stress incontinence is another characteristic symptom. (This is not to be confused with the frequency of urination normally experienced in the first and last three months of pregnancy, when the uterus is exerting pressure on the bladder and adjacent structures.*) The symptom is the involuntary escape of urine when you laugh, cough, sneeze, lift, run, and so on. You may wet yourself like this under conditions of stress, when the pressure on the pelvic floor is suddenly increased, but at other times urinary control is present. In severe cases, it may be difficult for the woman to make it to the bathroom, on arising, without dribbling or voiding on the way. Weak sphincters are unable to withstand the combination of gravity in the upright position and the pressure of a full bladder.

Sometimes urine leakage like this occurs during pregnancy and seems to clear up after the baby is born, but the basic weakness has manifested itself. Unless exercises are done postpartum to strengthen the muscles, the problem gets a little worse with each subsequent pregnancy, and recovery after each birth takes longer. Increasing age and decreasing hormones after menopause also hasten the process of deterioration. What begins as a lack of awareness or lack of conscious control becomes compounded by weakness and injury through childbear-

* Mention should also be made of female ejaculation, involving fluid from glands near the urethra, which occurs as part of a normal and powerful sexual response in a small percentage of women. Sometimes these women, their partners, and also their doctors confuse this with urinary incontinence.

ing. Professor Ralph Benson of the University of Oregon estimates that at least 50 percent of women suffer from incontinence at some stage of their lives, and 20 percent of all gynecological surgery is done to correct this unfortunate problem.

We have only to think how often we laugh, sneeze, cough, lift, strain, and run, thus putting pressure on the pelvic floor. These muscles are obliged to work consistently, with intermittent stress, and at a mechanical disadvantage against the force of gravity. Yet how often do we draw up the hammock with our voluntary effort to counteract these effects? It's no wonder that over the years the floor and the organs that it is supposed to support become displaced. When a bed gets progressively softer and less supportive, we tighten the springs as far as we can and may eventually place a board under the mattress. Likewise, we must tighten our muscles in the pelvic floor (which can always be improved, unlike bed springs!). If we don't keep them supple and strong, they will stretch to their limits, and extraneous aids, such as a pessary or surgical repair, may be required.

Not all inefficiency of the pelvic floor is associated with the trauma of childbirth and not all childbirth is associated with inefficiency of the pelvic floor. The problems of leaking urine accompanying exertion or of discomfort from sagging or prolapse of internal organs, which are typical symptoms of pelvic floor malfunction, can be caused by other factors. The cause may be congenital. It may also be a result of injury or disease involving the nervous system or specific nerves. Sometimes these problems are due to the process of muscle and tissue degeneration that occurs with aging, especially after menopause, when hormones are deficient. While these problems are more common in women over forty who have borne children, they can also be found among adolescents and young mothers.

Frequently the predisposition to difficulty in urinary control relates back to infancy, when the muscles were developed before the nerves that supply them. There is no control of the pelvic floor until pathways are developed and connections established between the muscles and the central nervous system. Until this occurs (around eighteen months) the child's perineal muscles are in a relaxed or emptying position — so any early success at toilet-training must be seen as owing more to good luck than good management! When the circuits between the pelvic floor and the brain are complete, the child must then learn voluntary control and the customs of the culture. It is

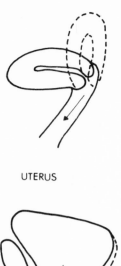

UTERUS

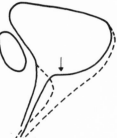

BLADDER

A well-defined angle is the key to stability.

thought that posture and other patterns of behavior in childhood account for this variation in neurological development, which in adulthood may be less than complete and thus results in problems that may persist or recur in pregnancy or later life.

The symptoms can often be alleviated by exercise, but at other times surgery is the only recourse. The pelvic organs that rely most heavily on support from below (the master sphincter) are the uterus and bladder. Both these organs are in their most desirable positions when the main body of the organ lies at a well-defined angle to its passage to the exterior. The uterus is very commonly "tipped" or retroverted — that is, angled backward instead of forward — but it is nevertheless positioned safely away from the vaginal canal.

Uterine prolapse is likely to happen when the uterus lines up with the vagina in such a way that it tends to slide down into this canal. Any increases in intra-abdominal pressure (such as straining on the toilet, prolonged standing, excessive stair-climbing, persistent coughing) will, in time, cause its progressive descent. Genital laxity can be prevented or minimized depending on the extent of obstetric trauma or the efficacy of exercise of the pelvic floor muscles before and after delivery.

When the internal bladder mechanism is impaired, the bladder wall becomes aligned with the urethral passage, as the uterus lines up with the birth canal. Loss of the angle at the neck of the bladder is beyond correction by efficient exercise alone, although functional and supportive muscle will enhance the success of the surgery. When urine escapes from this internal sphincter, the woman will typically try to hold it back with the external sphincter of the pelvic floor. This causes added stress and further weakness of the external sphincter. Re-education of the voluntary muscles is very necessary, although their deficiency may not be the primary problem. The angle at the back of the bladder may take years to become obliterated, so this, like most pelvic neuromuscular problems, is usually slow in onset, and early restorative exercise is very important in prevention or correction at the first sign of malfunction.

Leaking of urine, when it becomes a chronic problem in the adult, is even more embarrassing and depressing than vaginal herniation. The afflicted woman must cope with odor, skin irritation, and inflammation, which are aggravated by the need to wear absorbent pads.

Problems with the pelvic floor are so common that it seems that society just takes them for granted. Since at least half of the female population has some laxity of the pelvic floor with or without handicaps, doctors tend to think of the firm efficient perineum as the exception. It's not surprising, then, when doctors say (and believe), "What do you expect when you're forty-five and have had four kids?" These typical problems, which the general public "knows" about, provide basic standby material for comedians. Women's liberation movements, so busy with many fundamental issues, have not yet brought this topic into public awareness. Reports and confessions of these afflictions are still surrounded by shame, secrecy, and, for many, an acceptance that this is part of the hassle of childbearing. Articles on the subject are usually found in medical journals, where concern is with surgical rather than with preventive procedures, which could be initiated in the childbearing years or earlier. Issues of sex and birth control have a certain chic these days; urinary control problems, as yet, do not although they concern both sexes and are seen from childhood to old age.

However, there was one noteworthy exception. Arnold Kegel, a professor of obstetrics and gynecology at the University of California in Los Angeles in recent decades, did so much research in this field that in the United States his name has been given to the action of contracting the pelvic floor musculature: the Kegel exercise (see pages 35–38). His contribution to understanding and improving female pelvic function is unsurpassed and he achieved good results with muscle re-education in cases of urinary stress incontinence. Consequently, surgical correction of external sphincter weakness was discontinued at his clinic. Years after Kegel's pioneering work, however, postpartum restorative exercise is rare rather than routine, and the need for prevention is insufficiently emphasized. Part of the explanation is that most gynecologists are males — and surgical specialists. They also perform a creative stitch called the "husband's knot" when suturing the episiotomy, a surgical incision in the perineal tissue. This knot — an extra stitch or so — does not restore any pelvic floor function for the woman; it merely makes the vaginal entrance a little tighter. The name is significant since it reveals not only a male chauvinist bias but implies that the female vagina is quite passive and that improvements, therefore, need to be structural instead of functional. Her needs, as the name indicates, are secondary! Sometimes an actual tuck is taken as the surgeon attempts to sew up the birth canal outlet "as tight as a virgin" during the episiotomy or sometimes during later gynecological surgery.

This can cause real pain during sexual penetration. As long as doctors cling to an architect's view of the vagina, the value of exercise will be overlooked. Instead, surgical enlargement and closure of the opening for childbirth will continue, along with reconstruction in later life.

The Pelvic Floor in Pregnancy

As noted earlier, the pelvic floor must always support the organs and contents in the pelvic basin, but it performs this function at a structural disadvantage due to its design and a functional disadvantage caused by the usual neglect. The uterus, which is suspended between the bladder and bowel, relies particularly on pelvic floor support. It is not a fixed organ and the significance of its attachments by ligaments is minimal compared with support from below in maintaining its position in the pelvis. During pregnancy, the enlarging weight of the uterus creates additional, continuous, and increasing stress on the pelvic floor. It's like a shelf that bows if you put too many heavy things on it. So if the load factor cannot be altered, as it cannot be in pregnancy, then you must reinforce the floor. You can do this through exercise — in fact there is no other way to bolster it. Furthermore, hormonal effects cause the tissues to soften in preparation for delivery.

Pelvic floor exercises should be started immediately. While the learning process may be a little tedious, with practice the contractions become easier, and finally automatic and self-perpetuating. Consistent exercise of the pelvic floor is essential if you wish to avoid a whole chain of pelvic neuromuscular dysfunctions. Other benefits from this exercising that you will appreciate include, as we have noted, increased sexual enjoyment and relief from pelvic congestion due to the improvement in pelvic blood circulation.

The result of the increased pressure in pregnancy, together with infrequent muscle action in the supporting floor, slows down blood circulation and causes congestion in the perineum. Unless the pelvic floor gets occasional relief through changes in position and unless the pelvic floor muscles undergo active contractions, which pump the venous blood on its way, varicose veins in the vulva or, more typically, the rectum (hemorrhoids) may result. Toward the end of pregnancy, when the baby drops and the head engages in the pelvis, there is more compression of the pelvic organs and these symptoms are increased. Discomfort from such side effects is extremely common. Straining during elimination is always undesirable; it is particularly so during the maternity cycle, because of the stress on the abdominal muscles and pelvic floor. Constipation should be relieved with diet and exercise. Elimination may be made easier if the woman relaxes, with her feet supported on a stool, and allows the gentle interaction between abdominal compression and pelvic floor release. Contraction and relaxation of the pelvic floor stimulates bowel movement. The breath should be exhaled, not held. As in childbirth, forcing must give way to letting go, guided by the body's natural rhythms.

The Pelvic Floor in Labor and Delivery

The strong supportive role of the pelvic floor in pregnancy is temporarily relinquished during birth. The muscles need to relax, and all tension, which would slow the baby's progress through the birth canal, must be released. The pelvic floor is quite passive during the first stage of labor. In the second stage of labor it undergoes extreme distention to permit the delivery of the presenting part, usually the baby's head. After a pause the shoulders are delivered and the rest of the baby slides out. The delivery of the placenta then follows, after which further expansion of the vagina is no longer required.

Unlike the cervix, which over a period of many hours in the first stage of labor gradually and passively is thinned-out (effaced) and dilated, the vaginal canal has considerably less preparation for the passage of the baby. The outlet is forced to open very quickly in comparison with the cervix. Of course, the hormonal changes that have occurred in pregnancy make the birth canal softer and more elastic, so it expands and becomes very thin under the pressure of distention. This stretching causes the perineum to become numb, although until that point the sensations that accompany the stretching are described as "burning," "prickling," "pressure creating a desire to move the bowels," or "a build-up of tension like that before orgasm." The greatest stress, and subsequent stretching and/or tearing, is at the margins of the vagina, particularly near the anus in the back-lying position. An episiotomy is commonly cut here to enlarge the outlet and decrease the pull on the perineal tissues.

The advantages claimed for the episiotomy include minimizing stretching, preventing perineal tears, and reducing compression of the baby's head. It may shorten the second stage of

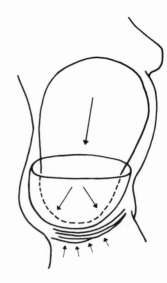

A large load leaves little room within the pelvic basin.

labor, when there is resistance from the pelvic floor. (The mother is tensing the muscles to counteract the pressure and stretching, withholding rather than releasing and *giving* birth). Episiotomies are also performed in instrumental deliveries and even when the mother has been given anesthesia, which results in total relaxation of the pelvic floor but eliminates her voluntary assistance in bearing down.

A midline incision is easier to repair and heals better, although some doctors are afraid of involving the anal sphincter and prefer to cut toward one side. In these cases there is more blood loss and greater postpartum discomfort. Muscle function is harder to regain when scar tissue forms on one side; the fibers have to reunite on the bias rather than in the central perineal body.

The low incidence of episiotomies in other countries, such as the Netherlands, shows that, while there will always be some complications where an episiotomy is necessary, such a measure need not be considered routine. There is always a chance of a perineal tear; no one's judgment is perfect. Doctors who perform episiotomies as a matter of course do so because they prefer not to take that risk. A first-degree tear should be regarded as acceptable since it heals spontaneously. Once the perineum is cut, however, the incision may be extended during the birth. Many physicians also feel that even if a tear were avoided the muscles would be irrevocably stretched. But it has never been demonstrated that routine episiotomies reduce damage to the pelvic floor structure. In fact, incision and repair may lead to poor anatomical results. Exercises to prepare and restore a stretched — but intact — perineum would seem more desirable. However, considering that most women neither present their obstetricians with an adequately supple, exercised pelvic floor that they can effectively release during birth nor assure their doctors that they know how to exercise these muscles postpartum, the doctors feel justified in taking a "preventive" step that women should have taken themselves.

The mother's acceptance of this intervention and the future results of the procedure are also most important. Sexual response, we have seen, can actually be marred because the vagina becomes too tight or too lax subsequent to surgical repair. Many women strongly dislike the thought of being deliberately cut, suffering stitches and perhaps scar tissue afterward. Episiotomy is also a major cause of blood loss. The intense concern that women feel about this intervention is revealed by the number of questions asked in childbirth education classes on this subject. It is minor surgery and informed consent by the mother should be required. It has also never been proven that episiotomies benefit the baby in any way, in the absence of fetal distress. It has even been suggested that the squeezing of the baby's chest by the intact perineum helps to expel mucus from its lungs.

Shaving of the lower pubic hair is less common now and done supposedly for the repair of the incision although no hair grows where the perineum is actually cut! Studies have shown that in women who have been shaved the incidence of infection is actually a little higher than in cases where the area is left untouched or the hair is just clipped with scissors so that razor nicks are avoided. Regrowth of the hair is also much more endurable when the hair has been cut rather than shaved. In countries where episiotomies are not the rule, women are not routinely "prepped."

Certain other factors can reduce the need for an episiotomy. If the second stage of labor is advancing rapidly, the side-lying position will eliminate the force of gravity and provide for a smoother control of the birth. If progress is slow in the second stage and there is difficulty with rotation of the baby's head, the need for intervention can be reduced by placing the mother in a propped position, thus making use of the force of gravity. If the baby's position is posterior, it often helps if the mother goes on all fours for a while, or lies sideways, with the back of the baby's head uppermost and the mother's upper knee drawn right up. It is essential for the mother not to pull on her legs nor should she push with her feet against resistance, since this creates muscular tension that spreads to the perineum. Teaching this unnecessary exertion is quite prevalent still, and an attendant will often put up siderails for the feet or encourage the mother to lift up her legs. During the second stage you should be loose from the waist down and your legs relaxed, spread apart, if half-lying. But it is most important that you choose a position that feels instinctively right. You may want to watch the crowning of the head or need guidance of the perineum from the attendant's hands. Massage and hot compresses may help, too, although some believe that it is better to leave the perineum alone and that the stretching sensations provide the best guide for breathing the baby out. But since birth is the culmination of pregnancy and labor, the way these are managed influences what trauma or intervention may occur. The expectant mother must psychologically want to "open up" her sexual organs. As during orgasm, there is a time when you must *let go* and trust in your body. The personality and physical and mental preparation of the mother are significant, but there are always a few factors outside anybody's control.

The Pelvic Floor in Postpartum

The vaginal outlet undergoes immense stretching during delivery, with or without an episiotomy. Stitches will cause discomfort for a few days until they are dissolved (or for the first 48 hours in the occasional cases when removable sutures are used). The muscles may be bruised and swollen, and the whole area tender to any pressure from thighs, buttocks, or internal strain from coughing, lifting, sneezing, and the like. During bowel movements support the sutured area with your fingers wrapped in tissues to minimize "fecal distress." Ultrasound (the type used by physical therapists, not the type used in obstetrical diagnosis) is a great help in relieving pain and in preventing scar tissue when the perineum is injured. Initially, attempts at muscle contraction of the pelvic floor immediately postpartum are met with dismay. You may feel absolutely nothing and perhaps have problems controlling urine for the first day or two. A reassuring fact, however, is that the vaginal sphincter is capable of amazing recuperation — if you recuperate it. If not, you will most probably join the majority of womankind, who suffer from some form of gynecological problems — laxity of the vaginal walls, bladder irritation or incomplete voiding, stress incontinence, constipation, painful intercourse, or other symptoms of pelvic dysfunction discussed on pages 24–28. Exercise must start at once before atrophy sets in.

If labor and delivery have gone smoothly, with only stretching of the pelvic floor, recovery will be easier. Under the force of distention there may have been tearing of the muscle sheet, or the nerve cells may be torn away from the muscles they supply. Sometimes the strain of delivery has caused the muscles to separate in the midline where they unite (diastasis, which can also occur in the abdominal muscles, see pages 58–60). Rarely, however, is the trauma so severe that exercise is of no benefit. Suturing alone, while restoring the structure of the pelvic floor, will not mean a return to function. You must exercise to make the muscles efficiently supportive again. The nerve connections to injured muscle fibers can be re-established with active exercise. This is the process of re-education.

Exercising the Pelvic Floor Prenatally

A great advantage is gained when a woman has sufficiently exercised her pelvic floor before delivery. There will be better support for the uterus and other pelvic organs during pregnancy, and greater relaxation during delivery because of the increased suppleness and control of the muscles. Muscle responds to the demands made upon it and progressive exercise increases the size and power of each muscle fiber. At the same time, the blood circulation becomes more extensive, so in the case of the perineum the muscles will be elastic enough to stretch over the baby's head with minimal damage to the muscle fibers through lack of oxygen and nutrients. Practice for release during the second stage should be done in a variety of delivery positions. By training the muscles before delivery, the mother knows better how to re-educate them afterward since she learned the exercise before the vaginal outlet was distended. She will be able to compare her present and past performances, and the comparison will increase her motivation to exercise postpartum. For this reason, pelvic floor exercises, above all others, should be included in a crash course or should be undertaken by the mother whose preparation comes so late in her pregnancy that other exercises would be of no value. A healthy exercised muscle will be restored much sooner than one that has been neglected and has only residual function after birth.

Exercising the Pelvic Floor Postpartum

It is never too late to learn how to contract the pelvic floor, and exercise is always of some value even if there is severe functional deficit. The process of learning is more difficult postpartum, when the muscles are stretched and slack, and feedback is poor.

Discomfort will be felt from the stitches but exercise will actually help to alleviate it. During muscle contraction, the edges of the incision will be pulled together rather than apart, so don't be afraid that the stitches will tear out. Be assured that this exercise is extremely beneficial no matter how sore you are or how scared you feel about doing it. Circulation to the wound will be increased; the blood brings fresh supplies of nutrients and carries off the accumulated waste products. Gentle muscle activity promotes healing in these ways, so you must not let the area stagnate. The same general benefits of exercise accrue as those from exercise before delivery. Circulation, which is usually sluggish in the postpartum phase, will be improved by pelvic floor contractions, and will relieve the pain not only of the episiotomy wound but of hemorrhoids or other varicose veins caused by pregnancy or labor and made swollen and tender by the pressure of delivery. Urine control improves, as does sexual participation. For this reason, some doctors recommend resumption of sexual intercourse after ten days, when the discharge (lochia) from the site of the placenta has ceased, instead of the usual six weeks. An episiotomy, if it has been done, is usually healed by the third week, but sensitive scar tissue may make intercourse painful. Comfort can be increased by tub baths, ice packs, infrared lamps, analgesic sprays and creams or lubrication ointment. The release technique learned for the passage of the baby through the birth canal is very useful during the first few attempts at sexual penetration.

The comfort aids for the episiotomy also minimize symptoms from hemorrhoids, although if you are using a heat lamp for the episiotomy, you may want to cover the hemorrhoid(s) with a gauze pad. In many cases these distended veins are caused by the pressure of delivery and will disappear postpartum. You can also try gently pushing them back inside with some lubrication while the hips are elevated. Remain in this position for a little while and perform some pelvic floor contractions to keep the anal sphincter tightly closed.

Exercise encourages the return of the muscle to its supportive role, which provides relief from the "low-down achy feeling" or the sensation that "everything is going to fall out." It also minimizes the likelihood of future pelvic problems. During the first few days, until the muscles resume their elasticity, you must consciously tighten the buttocks and sphincters and withdraw the pelvic floor each time you get up from the bed or a chair. This will avoid strain and the unpleasant sensations that accompany it, and the feeling of "spreading" you may have when you sit down.

If exercises are not done, the muscles will remain stretched and become further weakened as you resume your activities. Since muscles atrophy when they are not used, their eventual recovery will require more time and effort. By starting pelvic floor contractions immediately after birth, you will be doing them almost subconsciously by your six-week appointment.

Let your physician check and, it is hoped, confirm the success of your exercises at this time, rather than disappoint you with the news of your vaginal shortcomings.

Urination can cause difficulties in the immediate postpartum period. Once the compression from the uterus is no longer present, the stretch reflex of the bladder must adapt to the increased amount of room in the pelvis. This adjustment is complicated by the large amount of urine that accumulates after delivery because of the excretion of waste products from the uterus and from the general bodily activity involved in labor and delivery. The increased blood volume is also being reduced now that it is no longer needed. Voiding may be a problem (particularly after spinal or epidural anesthesia) and straining makes it worse. If the bladder becomes overdistended it may be necessary for the doctor or nurse to pass a catheter into the mother's bladder to empty the urine, but some simple measures you can take yourself may be of benefit. Try standing up or placing your feet on a stool when sitting on the toilet, or on a chair if you're using a bedpan. This will tilt the pelvis back so that the effect of gravity will assist you in voiding and the modified squatting position helps since there is compression of the abdominal cavity. Some deep breathing and pelvic floor contractions help to make up for the loss of intra-abdominal pressure and stimulate the bladder reflex. Gentle supporting pressure on the lower abdominal wall can also be tried, or turn on a tap so you hear water flowing. But remember — relax: do not strain.

It is quite usual not to feel the need for a bowel movement for several days after birth, particularly if an enema was administered. Again, stitches break down only if there is an infection or if there were simply not enough stitches, and it's better to find that out earlier than later. Avoid undue straining but do not be afraid to apply your usual abdominal pressure. Don't hold your breath — instead exhale slowly.

Technique for Pelvic Floor Contraction

The contraction of the pelvic floor is a subtle combination of several movements of several muscles. In addition, the muscles at the side of the pelvic floor move up and in toward the midline, which adds to the squeezing and lifting effect. The floor works as a unit, with tightening of the sphincters and elevation of the inside passages occurring together. Correct use of the muscles requires some understanding of how they are arranged and work, which is why there has been much elaboration on these points so far. Sphincters are rings of muscle which constrict; this happens also when you tightly close an eye. Feedback is also essential — your opinion as to how you are doing may be mistaken. In a class it is unlikely that the childbirth educator would check you, since this requires putting a finger inside your vagina, and it's impossible to tell merely by looking whether you're doing it correctly!

The pelvic floor muscles are contracted when you try to hold back a bowel movement or interrupt the urine flow, so this is one way to gain both awareness and control of these muscles. Stopping and starting the urine flow is an objective test of muscle power and can be done as an exercise to improve the strength of the pelvic floor. During this action, the front half of the muscular figure 8, which is the sphincter shared by both the urinary and vaginal passages, is worked strongly. It is this important sphincter that needs development — not the stronger anal sphincter. Although the sphincters work in coordination with the lifting of the pelvic floor, since the muscles unite in a key central area (the perineal body), it is possible with practice — and is essential — to emphasize the contribution of the front sphincter. It is easiest to concentrate on constriction of the vagina when there is something inside, particularly when you are first learning the art. You can check the muscle action yourself with one or two fingers; the bath is a clean and convenient place to make this investigation, or squat over a mirror.

Analogies with elimination are a common way to explain and encourage pelvic floor function. But it is more pleasant and just as effective to condition the birth canal and its supporting structures with "sexercises." Sex research has demonstrated the nature of sensation and response in the vagina. Unlike our fingertips, for example, which easily discriminate a pinprick, the stroke of cotton, and fine degrees of temperature, the vagina responds to deep touch, pressure, and stretch. This proprioception is also the way we get messages from other muscles in the body. Nature provides for increasing resistance to be encountered during intercourse by the engorgement of the tissues during sexual excitement. This building of the orgasmic platform decreases the amount of space in the vagina. The amount of stimulation felt relates to the extent of the orgasmic platform and the amount of resistance offered by the vaginal walls, which, although they are passively engorged, can be muscularly active.

Good pelvic floor muscles make the vagina snug and extra stimulation can be enjoyed by both partners during voluntary contractions of the vaginal sphincter. Sexual response here becomes conditioned with favorable experience, if the pelvic floor muscles adequately grip the penis.

The second trimester of pregnancy is the time when erotic interest is most intense. This is because the pelvic tissues are in a constantly engorged state similar to that which occurs during sexual arousal. This is an ideal time to work on your special exercise skills! Toward the end of pregnancy, there may be spotting of blood with intercourse or there may be other medical indications that cause your physician to advise against coitus at this time. But he or she should fully explain any prohibitions to both partners, lest they feel anxiety about the mother's or the baby's welfare. Unless sexual activity is contraindicated for medical reasons, there is no need to give it up, and considering that there will be, perhaps, several weeks postpartum when you may not feel like it, continue beforehand for as long as you wish.

One advantage of sharing the exercise in a sexual situation is the benefit of feedback and coaching that your partner can supply. In this way, the quality of pelvic floor contractions can be evaluated and improved. At first the contractions may be weak and fleeting, but as you persist they will become more pronounced and can be maintained for a few seconds longer. The muscles of the perineum are thin in comparison to such bulky muscles as the biceps and the muscle in the front of your thigh, which have great endurance and can be exercised repeatedly against resistance. The pelvic floor is more sheetlike, similar to the muscle that makes the front of the neck taut when we grimace. This enables it to become stretched and numb (more like a membrane than a muscle) during delivery, when it is under immense tension. Because of its special nature, the mixture of voluntary and involuntary muscle fibers and other types of tissue, its ability to sustain a series of strong or prolonged contractions is less than other muscles. Your partner can tell you how you are doing because your subjective interpretation may be unreliable. You may think that your seventh and eight muscle contractions were just as constricting as the first six, whereas your partner will feel if they started to fade away after, say, the fourth. You can also tune in to the sensations of slackness and release that naturally occur after orgasm since this is the ideal relaxed state of the birth canal, which you want to achieve during the second stage.

It is essential, then, given the fact that tolerance for strong and sustained contraction in the pelvic floor is only fair at the best of times, not to weaken it further when tolerance is very poor. Work within the number of contractions that you can do of equivalent strength plus one. If you try for ten in a row, you'll just fatigue the whole structure. As you improve, add an extra contraction before resting so that you slowly build up the series. (Ten is enough.) And avoid prolonged holding. It's tedious and tiring, like continuous standing, and is not the aim of the exercise. Frequent contracting and relaxing of the muscles is more beneficial, and fatigue is avoided by working within the inherent physiological limits.

Common Errors in Exercising the Pelvic Floor

Errors frequently observed include holding the breath and attempting to bear down, which strains the pelvic floor downward instead of drawing it upward. The abdominal and buttock muscles may also be tensed instead of the pelvic floor. It's all right to exercise the abdominal and buttock muscles at the same time, but you must take care not to substitute these muscles for the pelvic floor muscles.

Tensing of the inner thigh muscles at the expense of a pelvic floor contraction can occur as well. This usually happens when the exercise is taught in the ankles-crossed position. The beginner has difficulty discerning the sensation of perineal tightening when there is also tension from the much stronger muscles of the thigh, abdomen, or buttocks. Learning the exercise with ankles crossed can interfere with the comprehension of the specific action and its exact sensation. Furthermore, it may encourage an ineffectual remedy for real muscle weakness, as when the woman who experiences occasional urine leakage tries to hold it back by squeezing her thighs together. This extra effort in no way aids the weak sphincter. Control must be developed at the upper, most important, layer of the pelvic floor, which is placed at about the middle of the vaginal passage. To perceive the feeling accurately you need to practice with legs apart and think "high." Tensing crossed legs not only blurs sensation with the superfluous action of neighboring muscles, but causes you to squeeze lower, at the entrance of the birth canal.

Another common misconception is that assuming certain positions in which your legs are forced astride will stretch the pelvic floor. The positions most commonly claimed to achieve this are tailor-sitting, sitting with the soles of your feet pressed together, squatting, or sitting with your knees pulled up and apart toward your ears.

The pelvic floor is the supporting hammock of the pelvic basin only. It is not attached to the thigh bones in any way, therefore the position of the legs is quite irrelevant. The passage of the baby does stretch the pelvic floor — just as you do when you push your head through a tight sweater neckline. Stretching occurs at the circular margin of the opening, as it does at the vaginal outlet, regardless of the separation of the thighs (which therefore need not be as uncomfortably wide as is often the case when stirrups are used). The ability of the pelvic floor to stretch during the relatively brief phase of delivery is increased not by structural slackness but by its suppleness and elasticity, which means that it should be firm and supportive at all other times. Exercises before birth are designed to build up the pelvic floor muscles and their blood circulation; then more muscle fibers will survive under distention because the nerve and blood-circulation connections remain intact. Regeneration after childbirth is easier when the muscles are strong, not stretched, beforehand. The vagina is designed to distend naturally: it accommodates the penis during intercourse, and with the preparative softening of the tissues in pregnancy — the passage of the baby. It would not be desirable for the pelvic floor to become progressively stretched in pregnancy, as do the abdominal muscles. These undergo continuous stretching and do not get a chance to contract effectively until postpartum, when at first they seem like a worn-out elastic girdle. The only stretching of the pelvic floor that occurs is from internal stress; this can be prolonged stretching in the sense of weakening, when adequate support for the pelvic organs is lacking, or the distention of the birth canal that occurs during delivery. Anatomical facts preclude external stress, achieved by different body positions, from causing the floor to stretch. In fact, legs-astride positions would appear to have the opposite effect, for psychological reasons, since many women tense the pelvic floor when they feel "open" or "exposed." (Cultural conditioning is very strong here; girls learn to sit with their legs together or knees crossed.) Therefore it is good psychological preparation to practice pelvic floor release for delivery in these legs-astride positions. Furthermore, some of these positions are excellent for stretching other muscles, such as those of the inner thighs and the calves.

Learning Difficulties

Regular attempts to stop and start the urine flow usually teach the correct action, reinforce the specific sensation so that the muscles can be contracted the same way at other times, and provide an objective test to measure how effectively you interrupt the flow. But some women do not have sufficient muscle strength even to slow down the flow; they usually also have problems starting and finishing. It merely adds to their despair if their gynecologist cheerfully tells them to practice stopping and starting in order to strengthen the muscles. This solution is actually their fundamental problem! Attempting to work weakened muscles in this way with a full bladder can cause further anxiety, stress, and loss of control. Such women require special help to elicit and develop the correct muscle action.

Contractions must be done a few at a time but often, and without prolonged holding, as in any pelvic floor exercise. A pelvic floor that is undergoing re-education must be treated with care at all times. Make sure that you brace the muscles before lifting, straining, coughing, and so on. If you are experiencing a problem making it to the bathroom in the middle of the night or on arising, it will help to do a few pelvic floor contractions before you stand up and attempt to put pressure on the muscles.

You and your partner can practice and check vaginal sphincter contractions in the following ways:

1. Lying down should be tried first; the force of gravity is considerable when the muscle floor is weak. If muscle response is still lacking, try using gravity to assist, and

2. **Raise hips and buttocks on several pillows** (lying either on front or back) so that the pelvic floor tends to sink downward into your body, becoming closer to the pelvic base and the organs it supports. This is a reverse way of passively approaching a lifted position. Inverted yoga postures achieve this, but beginners should not attempt head and shoulder stands during the childbearing year.

3. Treatment may be sought from a physical therapist special-

izing in obstretrics and gynecology.* This may involve electrical stimulation of the muscles or, more commonly, use of a bio-feedback device. Because attempts to bear down, strain, or tense other muscles will not register a score, you learn the correct, isolated action of vaginal constriction. Once a woman learns to identify the pelvic floor muscles, increased awareness and function are readily developed. Diminishing scores indicate that muscles are fatigued from too many contractions or insufficient rest intervals. It is very encouraging to see the higher scores that you reach as you become able to contract the muscles more strongly. Such motivation is very important when there are learning difficulties, poor results at the start of the exercise program, or a feeling of hopelessness. (Despair leads to haphazard rather than consistent efforts. The success of exercise depends on repetition and regularity.)

Pelvic Floor Exercises

All the following activities concern the action of raising the pelvic floor and tightening the sphincters. Since these exercises involve lifting up and drawing in the muscles, they are not only safe but absolutely essential to do. Exercises 1 and 3 also teach you to recognize the lower position of the relaxed pelvic floor and the additional sensation of voluntary release, in preparation for the second stage of labor.

EXERCISE 1: CONTRACT AND RELEASE

Position: Lying down on back, side, or front. (On the front is the most comfortable position postpartum if you have had stitches.) Legs apart and chest relaxed for normal breathing.

Action: Draw up the pelvic floor, feel the additional squeeze from the sides as the sphincters are tightened and the inside passages become tense. Concentrate particularly on the front portion of the pelvic floor — the master sphincter surrounding the vagina and urethra. Place one hand over the pubic bones and think about tightening the birth canal as high as the level of your hand.

* See Resources.

Hold for two to three seconds and then completely relax. Note the sensation as the pelvic floor lets down loosely. Try to slacken it a little more, releasing any residual tension. (This is what you must be able to do during delivery.)

Do only 2 or 3 in succession before resting for a couple of minutes, and always end with a contraction to return the muscle floor to its supportive resting state.

Progression: Other positions — sitting, standing, squatting. When you have mastered the correct action, you can try combining and alternating pelvic floor contractions with those of neighboring muscle groups, such as buttocks, inner thighs, and abdominals, to test your awareness of control. Try to hold the pelvic floor for 5 seconds before relaxing. Try to do 5 contractions in a series before resting. Further progression of holding time or increasing the number in a series is not required; rather you can provide effective exercise of the muscle by doing this frequently, 50 times or more a day, in a series of 5, holding each contraction for 5 seconds. This way you don't get bored, or risk muscle fatigue by prolonged holding or frequent repetition without resting. Remember the physiological limitations of the pelvic floor!

EXERCISE 2: SEXERCISES

Position: Your choice, but some form of coital connection with the legs spread and relaxed.

Action: Grip the penis as firmly as you can with your vagina and hold for a couple of seconds before relaxing. Don't make any distracting movements and try to avoid tensing the buttocks and abdominals. Instead, focus on the sensation of the circular vaginal wall constricting. Repeat a few times until your partner feels that the strength of the contractions is diminishing. Rest and try again in a few minutes.

During this pleasant exercise the man does not need to exert himself at all, although he will probably feel stimulated to make small adjustments of penetration in order to coordinate with your muscle contractions. This, in turn, will encourage your muscle action, providing for greater mutual pleasure. With practice, vaginal sexual response can be conditioned so that orgasm occurs without direct clitoral stimulation.

Progression: This exercise provides for progressive increase in muscle strength as you learn to make the contractions stronger, more consistent, and more numerous. Remember to note the sensations of postorgasmic release in the birth canal muscles.

EXERCISE 3: THE ELEVATOR

Position: Any position, although one that eliminates the force of gravity, such as lying down, is easier at first.

Action: Imagine that you are riding in an elevator. As you ascend to each floor, try to draw up the perineal muscles a little more. Don't lose any of the tension that you have been progressively accumulating. Make it a smooth ride, as in modern elevators! When you reach your limit, *don't just let go!* You must descend, floor by floor again, gradually relaxing the muscles in stages. When you arrive at the basement — the resting level of tension in the pelvic floor — think "release." Try to slacken the perineum a little more so that you feel the finer degrees of muscle tension release.

Blow out through pursed lips so that you are increasing the intra-abdominal pressure. Feel that there is no strain on the pelvic floor below because air is being released from above. During second stage you want this to happen as you breathe the baby out with no tension in the pelvic floor muscles. Holding your breath to push creates a closed pressure area, like a balloon, and the sphincters automatically tighten as a protective reflex. This must be avoided — keep breathing, stay loose.

The exercise is completed with the muscles drawn into the uplifted or "ground floor level" position. As Sheila Kitzinger, the British author who popularized this exercise, says, you wouldn't walk around with your jaw hanging loose! Put a smile on your pelvic floor!

EXERCISE 4: THE FAUCET

Position: Seated on the lavatory, legs spread well apart for urination. Feet may be supported on a stool if commencing voiding is difficult.

Action: During urination, stop and start the flow a few times. Break it off smoothly with no dribbling.

Progression: Let a smaller amount pass each time! Take care not to increase stress and weakness if this exercise is too difficult (see pages 24–25). You may find this a tedious exercise, but it is a useful check of muscle power. At least, always concentrate on a strong uplifting contraction of the floor after any elimination. This will provide frequent opportunities for muscle exercise and serve as a reminder.

Aids: Let some urine out before exercising. Do not do this exercise during your first morning urination, when your bladder is very full, or at night, when you may be very tired and uncomfortable.

Opportunities Unlimited for Pelvic Contractions

Pelvic floor contractions are entirely private and can be performed at any time and in any place or position that you fancy, such as:

- During pelvic-tilting exercises (page 67).
- During bridging exercises (page 115).
- At red traffic lights.
- During boring parties.
- While stirring things on the stove.
- When you squat.
- During commercials on TV.
- Anytime you have to wait (especially standing).
- While brushing your teeth.
- When coughing, sneezing, laughing, lifting, climbing stairs, straining.
- Or any other time that you think of doing them.

Remember: Quality is more important than quantity. Slowly contract the muscles as you would in making a hard fist, not just closing your fingers but clenching to bring in every muscle fiber. About 5 in a series, holding each contraction for about 5 seconds — then rest a while. Always end with an uplifting contraction. Fifty a day, at least, during pregnancy and postpartum. Fifty a day, at least, *for the rest of your life.*

3 The Abdominal Muscles

IN CONTRAST TO the pelvic floor, the abdominal wall is something that we always notice in ourselves and others. The state of these conspicuous muscles is readily observable through our clothes, whether there's a trim waist to be admired or a "spare tire" to be disguised. Concern is usually more with appearance than performance, since the personal features of one's abdominal area significantly determine the size and type of clothing that we select. Many people are not aware of the role of the abdominal muscles in supporting the pelvis and lumbar spine and it may seem strange that muscles placed in front may relate to discomfort or pain felt in the lower back region.

The outward signs of the effects of pregnancy on the abdominal wall may be obvious, and while stretch marks, if they occur, will remain, there is no need for muscle weakness to persist as a permanent reminder. Most people will be familiar with some kind of abdominal exercises, but certain modifications and precautions are required during the childbearing year. Furthermore, a defect can arise in the supporting muscle structure or it may have occurred during a former pregnancy. This should be checked before starting abdominal exercises.

Structure of the Abdominal Muscles

Arranged like an extensive four-way corset, the abdominal muscles span the front of the trunk from the breastbone and ribs to the pubic bones, and around the side of the pelvic ridge that you can feel at each hip. Their arrangement and attachments are quite complex, but we can compare them to an elaborate corset. (Foundation-garment designers obviously took their model from nature.) The extensive diagonal fabric around the sides of a corset or girdle is similar to the two oblique abdominal muscles that overlap in such a way that each layer pulls in the opposite direction. The vertical panel down the corset's center represents the straight abdominal muscles (which are actually *two* recti muscles joining in the midline — an important point

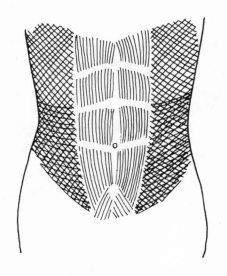

The abdominal muscles are like an elaborate corset.

that will be discussed later). An extensive horizontal waistband is formed by the transverse abdominal muscles.

Function of the Abdominal Muscles

Although each segment of the abdominal corset makes a key contribution, during exercises and activities the different parts are combined rather than isolated. For example, the top half of the corset is emphasized during movements with the upper trunk; the lower abdominals work to stabilize the pelvis when the legs are moved. The functions of the abdominal muscles are varied and they are:

- To maintain the proper positions of the abdominal and pelvic organs (including the enlarging uterus in pregnancy).
- To assist in deliberate breathing, singing, shouting, coughing, sneezing, vomiting, straining, elimination, and the second stage of labor.
- To control the tilt of the pelvis. The downward pull of the buttock muscles, together with the upward pull of the abdominals, maintains the correct alignment of the pelvis in relation to the backbone. The sideways pelvic tilt — hip-hiking — is also abdominal muscle action.
- To flex the trunk to one side, which involves half of the muscles at a time.
- To raise the trunk upward from a back-lying or semi-lying position. Commencing the movement is the most difficult part since the force of gravity must be overcome. Even just raising the head will cause the abdominal muscles to tighten.
- To rotate the trunk; for example, bringing one shoulder toward the opposite hip, or moving the hips in relation to the chest.
- To brace the body when it is under stress — lifting, straining, or outside blows. This is a reflex protection during effort.
- To stabilize the lower back during leg-raising, knee-rolling.

Our habitual use of the standing and sitting positions provides little stimulus for the abdominal muscles, nor are these muscles exercised when we walk at a normal pace on level ground. Therefore, the abdominals are usually the weakest group of muscles among the general population and their weakness is one of the most common causes of backache. Their maximal exertion occurs only when they must perform against resistance factors such as leverage and body weight, during trunk or leg raising and lowering from the horizontal, and while running, lifting, and so on.

The Abdominal Muscles During Pregnancy

In order to accommodate the increasing size of the uterus, the abdominal muscles permit an enormous degree of stretching. Evidence of this is also seen superficially by stretch marks, which indicate that the skin has reached the limit of its elasticity, and obliteration of the navel, which occurs around the seventh month. During pregnancy it is necessary to keep the muscles in good shape so that they can adequately support the load in front, which is placing increasing stress on the backbone. A correct pelvic tilt is the keystone. Without it, poor posture, muscle strain, and backache result. The abdominal muscles feel deceivingly fit during pregnancy because they are being continuously stretched over the enlarging uterus — the resistance keeps them taut. Because they are stretched so tight, it is important to avoid any positions or exercises that cause further stretch, or the muscles will be weakened.

It is understandable that without special effort on the mother's part after delivery, there will not be a complete return to former tone and length. The abdominal wall will still resemble a girdle, but one that is worn out or made of cheap elastic! Muscles, unlike girdles, do recover their inherent properties, and exercise during pregnancy will facilitate recovery afterward. Supple muscles, which have maintained their contractile ability and blood circulation as much as possible, will lengthen more easily and shorten more quickly afterward.

Many women are not interested in special exercises until they look and feel quite pregnant; then they are motivated to take action. There are a few reasons why prenatal exercises receive little emphasis in most childbirth preparation classes. The number of students may be large, the schedule very tight, the focus usually on preparation for labor and delivery. And frequently the expectant mother seeking advice or instruction is well into the last trimester. While it would be unwise to begin progressive abdominal muscle exercises at this time, certainly the essential exercises can and should be done. These maintain existing strength and firm the muscles. Any position or exercise causing extremes of movement, muscle strain, or stress on the joints, which are vulnerable because of the slackened ligaments, is most definitely to be avoided.

The Abdominal Muscles During the First Stage of Labor

The abdominal muscles should be completely relaxed for as long as possible during the first stage of labor. This permits the uterus to tip forward a little with each contraction instead of being restrained. Loose abdominals allow deep, slow breathing, and the gentle rising and falling of the abdominal wall shows that you are not voluntarily constricting the muscles as a result of tension. (This must be distinguished from forceful protrusion and retraction of the abdominal wall taught in the past.) When we are fearful or anxious, our mental state causes physical tension, with a consequent change in muscle state and in respiration. General relaxation, and particularly relaxation of the abdominal wall in the first stage, is therefore important in order for the mother to avoid unnecessary and interfering tension. Later in labor, however, voluntary relaxation of the abdominal wall during intensely strong contractions may become impossible. The breathing becomes lighter and automatically moves up into the chest at this time.

Transition: The uterus does not change from dilating to expulsive contractions like the flick of a light switch. On the contrary, this progress is often a stormy time, with contractions the longest and strongest of all and the mother feeling crosscurrents of sensation. Often there is a premature urge to push. A general rule is that pushing should always be withheld until dilation is complete (that is, 10 cms, or 5 fingers' measurement). But occasionally, when just a partial "lip" of cervix persists, or when the attendant wants to encourage descent of the baby along with the final degrees of dilation, he or she may advise *gentle* pushing for comfort along with the contractions if the urge is very strong. It would be rare for a laboring woman to be left alone without guidance at this crucial time, and, as each labor is different, the doctor or midwife must decide on the spot whether pushing is the appropriate response or whether this would risk injury to the cervix. In the latter case, breathing and distraction techniques must be employed to postpone the bearing-down for a little longer.

The Abdominal Muscles During the Second Stage of Labor

The first stage of labor involved the dilation of the cervix until its complete opening permitted the baby to exit. Until this point, then, the baby has not moved but has remained in the uterus during the many hours while the muscle contracted and shortened to pull the cervix open. The second stage of labor occurs when the baby moves down the birth canal, now pushed along by the expulsive contractions of the uterus and the mother's bearing-down efforts. This culminates in delivery.

The second stage is the exciting part of labor! The baby is, at last, on the way, and you can take an active role, which gives you a much needed psychological boost and a new wave of enthusiasm after the long hours of first-stage labor.

Position: While it is convenient for the obstetrician, particularly if an instrumental delivery is intended, the common practice of placing women on their backs for the second stage is most undesirable for many reasons. Compression of the major blood vessels between the uterus (especially during contractions) and the backbone interferes with circulation and blood pressure. The strength of the contractions may be diminished by as much as a third, and ventilation of the lungs is hampered. The need for obstetrical intervention is increased since it is so difficult to coordinate the bearing-down and birth canal release in this dysfunctional position. Women placed supine will invariable arch their backs and necks, straining rather than contracting the abdominal muscles. Furthermore, you want to watch the birth, not the ceiling! When left to choose for themselves — in other societies or during home births — women select a variety of positions that commonly include squatting, kneeling, or being on all fours. Birthing chairs support women in a sitting position and utilize the force of gravity. Beanbag chairs, common furniture in alternative birth centers, also prop the laboring mother in a functional and comfortable position.

The back-lying position has become modified in recent times. Ideally, you will be in a comfortable half-lying or propped position, with legs bent and relaxed apart, so that you are not fighting gravity. Side-lying may be preferred when the baby's progress is rapid since gravity is eliminated, pushing a little easier to withhold, and the pelvic floor under less stress. Among the advantages of both these positions are (1) that the back is supported and rounded, *c*-like, to conform with the passage of the baby, and (2) that you can remain relaxed below the abdomen. It is quite pointless to take on the additional task in labor of raising the head and neck — *against gravity* — for each push. If you are unfortunate enough to be lying flat on your back, this is unavoidable.

Although it is often taught, it is a waste of energy to pull up on your legs, as is illustrated in the drawing opposite. This results in unnecessary lifting of both upper and lower limbs. Such heavy exertion would not even be taught in a prenatal exercise class. This extra work is not required if you are sufficiently propped and can relax your legs. A restful position of comfort avoids the need to rock up and down on your spine for pushing, which can result in considerable backache. Some women prefer to actually extend their bodies during labor, instead of being flexed into a ball. Birth is more a matter of letting go than mustering force and only the woman herself knows what feels right.

When you rest between contractions, stretch out your legs and move your knees and feet. This is always possible in the labor bed, but if you change to a delivery table the legs are generally confined in stirrups. These overutilized devices are another feature of childbirth that indicates that the convenience of the physician is more important than the comfort and contribution of the mother. The height and distance between the stirrups can be adjusted, so do request adjustment if you are very uncomfortable, or ask if your legs can be just relaxed apart — as far as the delivery table permits!

Direction of the expulsive force: The baby's path is *down* the birth canal, *up* around the pubic bone, and then *out* into the world. So those who deliver when flat on their backs actually push *uphill*. If the mother is half-sitting, or lying on her side with a rounded back, this helps to bring the base of the pelvis well forward, which means it is tilted back in relation to the spine, providing a wider and more functional position for delivery. Gravity, as in squatting or kneeling, is a great help also. The push is directed vaginally, in front of the rectum — a difficult idea to follow when the baby is still in the uterus and when the urge to push is not present. Rehearsals should be done in various delivery positions so you feel free to seek your own style of birth.

Maternal Effort: Many people believe that childbirth is a major athletic event. Total exertion during labor thus justifies the exhaustion that is commonly experienced with this approach. Nevertheless, babies do get born, with or without special help from the mother or her attendant. Appropriate

Being propped from behind and released from below is preferable to the exertion of fighting gravity, lifting and tensing the lower limbs.

assistance is helpful and, of course, sometimes essential. However, time, timing, and relaxation are the most important considerations for second stage. Often there is a lull following complete dilatation, which is physiological and allows the mother to enjoy a rest. The urge to push is felt only when the head is low enough to stimulate the stretch receptors in the pelvic floor. Frequently, women are made to bear down before the uterus is ready, and an arbitrary time limit is set for delivery. This leads to the mother having to force the birth instead of allowing events to flow with their own rhythm. When the urge is irresistible, the mother spontaneously bears down. Only she experiences the inner cues. Many midwives feel that women cannot be taught how to push a baby out any more than one can be taught how to have an orgasm. At a certain point, the mind lets go and trusts in the physical response of the body. Physicians, however, are usually in a hurry and also want to actively "manage" the labor.

How much assistance from the mother's voluntary efforts is appropriate? It would seem logical that the informed, prepared mother is the best judge of this so that she can harmonize her response to the contractions just as she did in the first stage of labor. Expulsion is then controlled according to the variety and intensity of the contractions rather than forced on principle. Often, however, the mother is subject to a ceaseless chorus of those around her exhorting her to bear down, which does not allow for the differences felt from woman to woman and from contraction to contraction within the same individual. This point is well illustrated in a popular Lamaze birth film, where a domineering nurse (obviously very proud of her movie debut!) bellows incessantly, "PUSH PUSH PUSH PUSH PUSH PUSH PUSH PUSH PUSH . . ." Such well-intended direction is at worst defeating and at best distracting for the mother who is attempting to tune in to her uterus, which she may well trust more than she does an outsider. Pushing, of course, is very important in slow and difficult labors, but other factors play a role as well — such as the mother's position, which can help or hinder and may also affect the direction or "knack" of pushing. Relaxation may be all that is needed to let the uterus push the baby out. In occasional cases women report no urge to push. (Squatting or kneeling can be tried, and/or pressure on the pelvic floor from the attendant's finger(s) inside the vagina if there is no progress.) However, this is most often the result of medication; and obviously anesthesia, even epidurals, will interfere with the bearing-down reflex.

The key concepts for an ideal second stage involve confidence in one's physically healthy and active body combined with an ability to coordinate and relax groups of muscles, rather than the idea of maximal maternal effort. If the abdominal muscles are weak, part of the expulsive effort will be dispersed, and the force from above will be partly wasted if you do not release from below. Without relaxation of the pelvic floor, the passage of the head through the birth canal will be slower. This ability to release is much more important (though much less instinctive) than the exertion of pushing. But releasing and pushing are related in the sense that if there is much resistance from the birth canal, then more expulsive force will be necessary to overcome it.

The pelvic floor should automatically relax during bearing-down unless the breath is held. During elimination you can also observe the relationship between increasing the pressure within the abdomen on exhalation while at the same time releasing the pelvic floor muscles. Despite this reciprocal relationship, the unprepared and apprehensive mother, on feeling the enormous pressure on the pelvic tissues and the stretch of the distending vaginal outlet, becomes alarmed and tenses the pelvic floor instead of releasing it.

Psychological preparation is important for delivery: grasping the principles involved, understanding what can happen, what you might feel, and how you can help. If you take every opportunity around the house to assume such positions as tailor-sitting, squatting, and legs-astride, you may find it easier to relax during the delivery, when your bottom will be bared and your legs spread apart. Some women, swept along by the intensity of the physical events and the accompanying emotion, just couldn't care less about appearances, but there are others who feel ill at ease and are concerned about escape of contents from the bowel. Extreme rectal pressure, more uncomfortable than painful, may be felt at this time and for these reasons an enema is often given (although it is also used to stimulate labor). In any case, delivery of the baby is of greater significance than the state of the sheets!

Coordination of pushing with breathing is the other aspect and is essential if you are to avoid useless straining or prolonged breath-holding. Visible signs of straining include a red face, taut neck muscles, bloodshot eyes, and burst capillaries in the cheeks. Exertion with a closed glottis* results in severe cardiovascular effects. Blood pools in the veins of the legs and

* This is known as the Valsalva maneuver, after the seventeenth-century Italian physician who recommended this technique to expel pus from the middle ear.

pelvis because it cannot return to the heart against the extreme pressure in the chest. (This pooling is further aggravated with epidural anesthesia and the back-lying position.) Therefore blood pressure and output from the heart fall. Circulation and oxygenation are impaired and it takes only about 5 seconds for the fetal heart rate to drop. No wonder second stage is usually limited to one or two hours: could mother or fetus stand much more?

The closed pressure "balloon" that is formed during the period of strain distends the abdominal wall outward, which puts great stress on the recti muscles. Reflex tightening of the pelvic floor is unavoidable. This unnecessary forcing, often referred to as "leaning on the contraction," also strains the attachments of the pelvic organs. Interference with the circulation, through lack of venous return, predisposes to varicosities of the rectum and vulva. Prolonged breath-holding also causes the mother to gasp air suddenly when she reaches breakpoint. The resulting retraction of the abdominal muscles creates a suction pull, which tends to negate her effort. This causes the baby's head, which slips back and forth a little during the progress of second stage, to regress even further. Tiring and needless head movements often go along with this jerky pattern of pushing. Concentration on the inhaled breath leads to tension, and sometimes hyperventilation. On the other hand, there is always reserve air in the lungs to be exhaled. Strong expulsive urges may not give the mother time to first take in a breath. In spontaneous pushing, the air is audibly exhaled. The air escapes slowly and often noisily because the lips and glottis are partly open. Braking the breath in this way allows the ribs to stay firm and the diaphragm slowly ascends as the abdominal muscles are drawn in around the uterus. Indeed, if no sound is heard, this means that the breath is being held and the body will be tense. Following exhalation, the incoming air is physiologically regulated and the progress of the head is smooth. One or several pushes may be heard during a contraction, depending on the urge that is felt by the mother. Spontaneous pushes last only a few seconds, which is much shorter than when pushing is directed by an attendant.

Exhaling during birth is advised for the same reasons as during elimination, exercise, or any form of exertion. Respiration is maintained and fluctuations in blood pressure are avoided. The pressure within the abdomen is increased because the volume is diminished. The rib cage, diaphragm, and abdominal muscles all interact as a unit. The abdominal muscles shorten and pull inward as the air is forcefully exhaled. Traditionally, hospital staff have discouraged vocal expression of feeling during labor. The popularity of the "quiet" birth has also led to the inhibition of the mother's experience of birth, despite the good intentions of her attendants. In a recent British film, a mother is told "Shssh" when she ecstatically cries out as the baby is being born. Moans, grunts, and groans are the natural music of labor. Certainly untrained women achieve a balance of respiration in this way. The grunt that accompanies a karate chop or the wail let out by a javelin thrower are other examples of this. Divers exhale under water instead of holding their breath. Only if you can let the air go can you release tension, which allows the physiological flow of energy.

A general guideline for maternal effort in the second stage, then, is to push only when you absolutely cannot resist the urge to do so. It is a little like swimming breaststroke or treading water: there is a time for the abdominals to tense and a time for air to be exchanged. Working with the body like this instead of relentless pushing, allows the birth canal time to fully distend to accommodate the baby's head, and prevents undue maternal fatigue.

An alert woman with good abdominal muscles that she can effectively coordinate with the expulsive urge and pelvic floor release can exert a considerable amount of voluntary force to speed along the second stage. However, the amount of maternal effort required will depend on the particular circumstances of her labor. She must be guided from within. Sometimes the baby is moving very fast and the mother will be asked to refrain even from pushing. The attendant is the one watching the action at the other end, and as the birth approaches he or she helps judge how much assistance from the mother is needed.

Your partner can be most helpful at this time by repeating the doctor's words, since many women are totally absorbed in the events occurring inside them. If the baby is coming out really fast (and babies can, especially in second or subsequent births), you'll want to allow the pelvic floor as much time as possible to be stretched gently. At the moment of *crowning* you may hear a sudden command to "stop pushing" or, more positively, "pant." Now you must breathe out the baby's head or presenting part, just as you would ease your own head slowly through a tight neckline.

Until this moment, whenever the uterus rested between expulsive contractions, the head slipped back a little due to the resilience of the birth canal. As the baby emerges from the bony

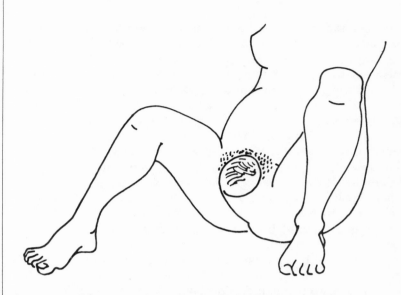

Pant, don't push, during crowning. Let the outlet slowly stretch.

pelvis, the back of the head extends beyond the mother's public bone and cannot slide back inside anymore. Next, the perineum must be finally negotiated as the head forces outward through the vagina. You will feel intense stretching and burning sensations, followed by a natural numbness. A calm, controlled delivery results in minimal trauma to the pelvic floor by allowing gradual distention — without tearing or episiotomy — of the birth canal.

It is essential that you understand the importance of refraining from a hearty push at the moment of birth — and prepare for it. This is difficult to do. You will have been pushing for perhaps quite a while, with encouragement from those around you; the uterus is still contracting expulsively; the next push will bring your baby into the world — yet you must let the uterus just nudge the baby out by itself. Simply "not to push" while experiencing the urge of the uterus is virtually impossible. Panting will help; it will not take away the urge but it aids you in controlling it. You blow the force outward instead of confining it inside. The diaphragm fluctuates, the ribs move, and, since the abdominals no longer have a firm base to work from, the power to push is greatly reduced. Usually you can observe the progress of events in the mirror above you, or you can feel the head with your hand. Some mothers become tired or the urge to push may not be strong and so the doctor will be coaxing each push all the way to the end.

Remember:

- Don't strain. Let go and flow with the contraction.
- Relax the pelvic floor throughout second stage. Don't tense the muscles when you feel rectal pressure, the vagina stretching, or the gaze of many eyes! Relax *all* sphincters and the mouth, too — with your lips slightly parted.
- Direct the push low down and in front — increase the pressure in your abdomen, not in your face! Don't strain so that you screw up your eyes — you might miss the moment of birth!
- Always take one or two deep breaths to refuel at the start and the end of a contraction. Exhale slowly as you bear down.
- Push only as long and hard as you feel the urge to do so. Avoid prolonged pushes, which affect your breathing, circulation, and also the baby's heart rate.
- When asked to refrain from pushing at any time — immediately relax the head back and pant. Keep it light and brisk — don't blow out hard and pull in the abdominals at this time.

The Abdominal Muscles Postpartum

The abdominal muscles are very loose and stretched after delivery and provide inadequate support for the pelvis and lower back. At this time these joints are particularly at risk because of the hormonal changes in pregnancy, which softened their protective ligaments. It is essential now to avoid any strain on the backbone or any stretching of the abdominal muscles. Exercises, then, are performed in stable positions where support is maximal and unnecessary effort avoided. The ligaments will gradually tighten back to their former stage as the uterus returns to normal, due to the physiological adjustments of the body during the postpartum weeks. Returning the abdominal muscles to their former shape, size, and efficiency, on the contrary, requires *your active input.* Best results are achieved when exercises are commenced *within twenty-four hours* after delivery.

Initially, you will be tensing, retracting, and pulling in the muscles to coax them back to their former length. Since the abdominal muscles have been subjected to prolonged tension stress, it is important not to overwork them at first but to repeat the exercises a few at a time and often. The exercises are simple and completely safe; they are easy to do and can be performed on the bed. Strong exercises must not be attempted until there has been good recovery of the abdominal wall and pelvic floor. This will vary with each woman and relates to her physical condition before pregnancy, her labor and delivery, and the management in the immediate postpartum phase.

Remember always to brace the pelvic floor — if you don't, your stitches will remind you to! Do not perform strong abdominal muscle exercises until you correct any lingering sphincter weakness, or until you have checked the state of the abdominal wall.

The key to success is *begin early, repeat often!*

Problems with the Abdominal Wall (Diastasis Recti)

After childbirth, the abdominal muscles are always stretched and slack. The waistline may be lost and the abdominal wall may continue to bulge later on if the transverse waistband muscle is weak. But a structural defect, which must be detected and corrected if present, can occur in the supporting corset. Most women after childbirth do have some degree of muscle separation.

If you look again at the diagram of the abdominal muscles (page 46), you will notice that there is a seam down the center of the front panel. Rather than one single band of muscle extending vertically along the midline of the abdomen, there are two halves — the right and left recti muscles. The corset is thinnest at this point since these broad flat bands form a single muscle layer, unlike the other abdominal muscles that overlap at the flanks. These recti muscles instead are lined and covered only by sheaths of fibrous connective tissue from the neighboring muscles, which unite in the central seam (the linea alba). This seam is about half an inch wide and with the cross seams also present can be readily observed in well-developed athletes when the abdominal muscles are tensed. During pregnancy, the superficial layer turns dark in some skin types and is then known as the linea nigra.

The hormones circulating in pregnancy cause this central seam to soften, along with other fibrous tissue changes. The abdominal muscles and their seams are expanded and stretched so that the body can accommodate the growing baby. Most of the weight of the uterus falls on the front wall of the abdomen, and the recti muscles in particular act to maintain intra-abdominal pressure under stress during any form of straining, in elimination, or undue bearing-down efforts in the second stage.

The umbilical or navel area is always potentially weak due to our early development since it originally was the sides of the embryo, and even in adults hernia can still occur at this point. The softening and stretching of the linea alba, which extends above and below the umbilicus, makes the central connection vulnerable. It is not uncommon for the recti muscles to separate — to be pulled away from their parallel union in the midline through stretching and straining of the muscles. It is just like a zipper, which has been closed, spreading open at the greatest point of stress. It is essential to realize that you may be unaware of this since you feel *no pain* from this condition directly (although you may have chronic backache).

This separation is frequently acquired during pregnancy. It may come on gradually (particularly with subsequent pregnancies) or result from sudden exertion imposed on underlying muscle weakness or other problems. The cause is a combination of the hormonal softening of tissue, the stretching of muscle, and excessive strain occurring in later pregnancy, when the muscles are in a lengthened state. One of the many reasons for avoiding double-leg–raising exercises is that they can cause or increase separation of the recti muscles. "Jack-knifing" from a horizontal position is also a danger.

Laxity and weakness of the abdominal muscles are conducive to their separation since strain during pregnancy or labor will be registered at the central junction, just as a seam in your clothes will split before the fabric. Other predisposing factors include obesity, multiple pregnancy, a large baby, excess fluid in the uterus, or a pendulous abdomen from former pregnancies. The condition is usually observed postpartum, although sometimes women or their physicians may pick this up in late pregnancy. Make sure that you investigate any bulging of the abdominal wall that you observe when getting out of bed or the bath. Separation of the recti muscles may occur during the second stage of labor, when prolonged breath-holding during pushing strains the recti muscles as they attempt to maintain pressure within the abdominal cavity. Straining during elimination, if habitual, is also a contributing factor. Learn to bear down gently (as if for the second stage!) and intermittently. Relax your legs with your feet on a stool and correct your diet

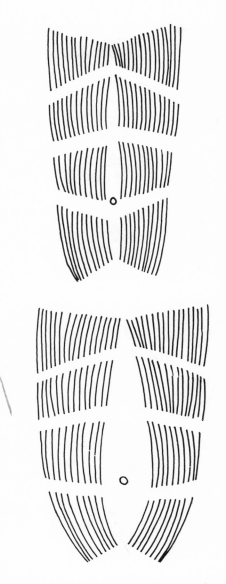

The recti muscles can separate as a zipper opens under stress.

to avoid constipation. General exercise will improve abdominal muscle support and intestinal activity which in turn help constipation.

The gaping of the muscles can be slight or so severe that the uterus or even abdominal contents can be felt protruding through the space. If not corrected, a state of muscle imbalance persists and the abdominal wall will remain weakened and will not be supportive for a subsequent pregnancy. Since the recti muscles are important in controlling the tilt of the pelvis, which in turn supports the backbone, their weakness can give rise to poor posture and pain in the lower back.

CHECK FOR SEPARATION OF THE RECTI MUSCLES IN PREGNANCY

During pregnancy it is important to recognize any separation, if it is present, in order to take care that further separation of the muscles is prevented. Do not do any type of curl-up or leg-lowering exercises if you have a separation of three fingers or more. All the other exercises in this book can be done safely. Use caution when changing positions, particularly when your trunk or legs are moved against the force of gravity. Always roll to your side before sitting up.

A check for separation can be done at any time during pregnancy if you suspect a split in the central seam. In the early months, before structural changes have occurred, check for a gap, as in the postpartum phase, instead of a bulge. For the last three months, do the investigation as follows:

Position: Lying on your back, knees bent.

Action: Slowly raise your head and shoulders until your neck is about 8 inches from the horizontal. Your chin should be tucked in and arms stretched out in front.

Check: A bulge in the central abdominal area is usually observed when the muscles have parted. If in doubt, you can feel if there is a softer region more than an inch or so in width between the taut recti muscles on each side. Check how many fingers you can insert horizontally in the gap.

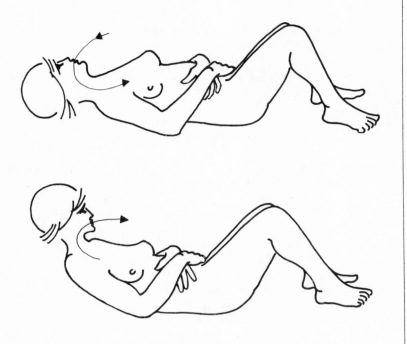

Support the recti muscles as you raise your head on outward breath.

Special Exercise for Separated Recti Muscles in Pregnancy

Position: Lying on your back, knees bent. Cross your hands over the abdominal area so that you will be able to support the two muscles as you raise your head.

Action: Breathe in deeply. As you slowly exhale, raise your head forward to your chest until just before the point at which the bulging between the muscles appears. Keep your shoulders on the floor. Return slowly to the starting position. If your abdomen is very obese, it may be necessary to support the recti muscles with your wrists and to cup your hands, one above the other, to confine the central bulge.

This exercise should be done a few times, when lying on the bed in the morning and the evening, so that the recti muscles can be kept in maximum tone and to discourage further separation.

CHECK FOR SEPARATION OF THE RECTI MUSCLES IN POSTPARTUM

A postpartum check for separation of the recti muscles is done around the third day after delivery. Until this time the whole abdominal area feels so slack that the test is not reliable. Besides, you will already have had two days of graded exercises to prepare you for the extra work in closing the gap, if required.

Position: Lying on your back, knees bent. Press the fingers of one hand firmly into the area around the navel.

Action: Slowly raise your head and shoulders until your neck is about 8 inches from the bed. You will feel the bands of muscle on each side pull toward the midline, pushing your fingers out of the way.

Check: How many fingers remain in the gap? A slight gap, 1 or 2 fingers wide, is just tissue slackness and will tighten of its own accord. But if you can place 3 or 4 or more fingers between the taut bands of muscle, then you need to make a special effort to restore the integrity of this area.

Special Exercise for Separated Recti Muscles in Postpartum

Position: Lying on your back, knees bent. Cross your hands over the abdominal area so that you will be able to pull the muscles toward the midline as you raise your head.

Action: Take in a deep breath: As you slowly exhale, raise just your head off the bed at the same time pulling the underlying muscles together with your hands. Return slowly to the horizontal.

Raising just the head activates only the recti muscles. As they become stronger, you must be able to raise your shoulders off the horizontal, which brings in the other abdominal muscles. These muscles insert into the central seam, so the movement must be done slowly in order for the recti muscles to stay aligned when these neighboring muscles exert their pull as well. Do not add your shoulders to the load until the recti muscles can cope with a head raise, without being supported.

Raising your head and shoulders on *outward* breath forces the muscles to work without the fixation of the diaphragm, since it moves up in the chest, emptying the air. If you were to hold your breath, the diaphragm would move down and increase the pressure inside the abdomen. When the muscles are weak, they are unable to compress the abdominal wall if pressure within is increased, so they bulge outward. *Bulging must be avoided at all times* by consciously contracting the abdominal muscles when any strain is likely and by performing these exercises on exhaled breath.

To encourage the recti muscles to resume their midline position, repeat the special exercise often, at least 50 times a day. Do 10 each hour if you can. Remember to do them slowly and to take a rest when you need it. Each day improvement will be noted if you are conscientious, and the gap should be closed back to the normal half-inch within a week or so. If you do the exercise less consistently it will take longer.

Until you have closed the gap, avoid exercises that rotate your trunk or twist your hips or bend the trunk to one side. Since the other abdominal muscles are indirectly attached to the recti, there will be muscle imbalance, which will pull them apart. Some separation may return after progressing to curl-ups if the recti muscles are not yet strong enough and need more work. Keep checking and appreciate the interaction of the whole abdominal corset.

Important Principles For Abdominal Muscle Exercises

Toward the end of pregnancy and the early postpartum, you perform the same essential exercises. It is logical that the muscles you prepare are the ones you will restore later and it is easy for you to remember the program if you practiced it in pregnancy.

The starting positions and actions of the following exercises are chosen to prevent strain on joints or muscles. Most of the exercises emphasize control of the pelvic tilt since this improves posture and relieves back strain. These movements require minimal exertion and help to maintain the condition of the muscles as they expand over the enlarging uterus. Some degree of progression is naturally provided since the muscles work harder as the weight of the uterus increases.

However, stronger exercises that progress the abdominal muscles against the resistance of gravity are required to *improve* the condition and power of the muscular corset. Exercise in pregnancy or even before should be commenced as early as possible so that you have achieved the minimum normal strength levels before the muscles start to stretch. Progressions that enable you to pass the basic tests and to advance to optimum strength are described at the end of the chapter.

Abdominal muscle exercises using leverage and the force of gravity for resistance are typically activities which involve the raising and lowering of the trunk or the legs. Sit-ups emphasize action in the upper part of the abdominal corset as the muscles shorten to raise the trunk. Leg movements involve strong stabilizing work from the lower abdominal muscles to control the pelvic tilt. It is not easy to properly strengthen the abdominal muscles because their action is complicated by an associated group of muscles — the hip flexors. Double-leg–raising (see Chapter 1, page 17) and the conventional sit-ups with the legs out straight are commonly used to achieve this goal, but evidence shows that they are undesirable as well as often ineffective. Many a person is proud of his or her ability to do a series of sit-ups or leg-raises; however these actions depend largely on the hip flexors and frequently give rise to back pain because they pull on joints of the lumbar spine.

The key to good abdominal exercises is to protect the lower back from the adverse pull of the hip flexors and to be in control of the leverage and resistance from gravity. The exercise of raising and lowering the outstretched legs, we have seen, is potentially dangerous to the spinal joints. It should be modified so that the knees are bent and the heels can be rested on the surface at any time when the back threatens to arch.

These points are important when performing sit-ups:

1. *Always check for a diastasis of the recti muscles* (pages 61–62).

2. *Postpone any exercises that cause you to feel strain on the pelvic floor.* Work more on pelvic floor contractions until the pressure of stronger abdominal action can be withstood.

3. *The knees should be bent.* This flattens and mechanically protects the lower back. Never do double-leg–raising.

4. *Half-way is enough.* The abdominal muscles raise the trunk from the horizontal to an angle of about 45°, after which the hip flexors take over and complete the movement. Just curling up 7 or 8 inches, letting your waist remain on the surface, is sufficient to exercise the abdominal muscles.

5. *The feet should not be held down.* This encourages the contribution from the hip flexors and may obscure weakness of the

actual abdominal muscles. When these muscles are strong, it makes little difference whether the feet are stabilized or not.

6. *Diagonal movements should be performed as well as straight up and down.* This ensures that all portions of the muscular corset are exercised.

7. *The movement must be a smooth roll, with the pelvis tilted back and the chin tucked under.* Jerking must be avoided and the back should never be held straight, as this favors hip flexor action.

8. *Never hold your breath, exhale on exertion.* The abdominal muscles should be pulled *in* as you breathe *out:* bellybutton toward backbone.

9. *Remember the gradual warm-up and cool-off.*

For many people, the action of curling up while lying flat is impossible to commence. The initial raising of the head and shoulders is the most difficult part of movement, as the average under-exercised person knows only too well! The effects of gravity are greatest as you leave the horizontal and the abdominal muscles must contract from a lengthened state. Preliminary strengthening exercises help you achieve the ability to do a curl-up with careful gradations so that you avoid strain, jerking, or the need to fix your feet. You start from a point where

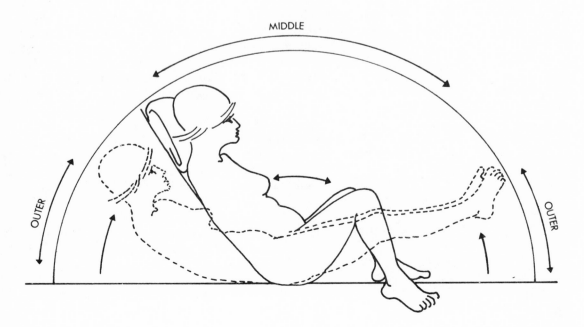

there is *least* effect of gravity and work back down from the knees. Most muscle activity normally occurs in middle range; that is why outer range movement such as raising the trunk or the legs is felt to be major effort.

The muscles contract with less effort when they are placed in a shortened position. You progress from the easy part of the movement to the more difficult. Trunk lowering is just a little easier than trunk raising, so you start close to your knees and then, allowing the abdominal muscles to lengthen as you roll back a little — then contract them as you sit up again. You move back and forth within the limit of your control. As your strength improves you will be able to move further back to the horizontal, taking on more resistance from gravity until you can sufficiently match it in order to execute a curl-up. In the beginning, stretch your arms out in front for extra assistance to counterbalance the trunk.

It is desirable that you achieve this minimal level of strength so that you can bear down with contractions as required in second stage. Furthermore, if you happen to be inadequately propped for this pushing phase, you will actually have to perform a series of curl-ups as you attempt to coordinate your effort with the contractions. If second stage lasts for an hour or so, and it often does with first babies, it is no wonder that the mother becomes extremely tired and often suffers backache for a long time afterward.

If you are well into the last trimester and have not been exercising the abdominal muscles, save the curl-ups for your postpartum program. If you cannot readily perform a movement, then you must not exert undue strain. In any case, during the last few weeks of pregnancy the size of the baby gets in the way. The other exercises will maintain existing strength at this time and can be done with ease and comfort.

EXERCISE 1: ABDOMINAL-TIGHTENING ON OUTWARD BREATH.

This exercise combines deep breathing with abdominal muscle work.

Position: Lying on back or side, knees bent. Place hands on abdominal area below ribs (for the learning process; they can be removed later).

Tighten the abdominal muscles on the outward breath.

Action: Take a deep complete breath in through the nose, feeling the nostrils widen slightly. Breathing through the nose warms and filters the air. Keep the ribs as still as you can and let the abdominal wall expand upward. Then, lips slightly parted, blow the air out through the mouth slowly but forcibly, pulling in your abdominal muscles all the while until you feel you have completely emptied your lungs. It's like sustaining a note while blowing a trumpet or singing.

Progression: Other positions, such as sitting or standing. Avoid taking too many deep breaths in succession — you may get dizzy. Deep breathing is very important in pregnancy and the early postartum phase, but at other times this exercise can be done as simple abdominal muscle contractions, on normal outward breath in standing, sitting, or other positions. A rocking chair is ideal! This works the transverse muscles, which compress the abdominal contents and prevent the abdominal wall from bulging. Repeating this now and then — for the rest of your life — keeps the muscles in tone.

EXERCISE 2: PELVIC-TILTING

This exercise is a favorite activity for improving posture and relieving backache and stiffness, at any time of life as well as during childbearing. It works the abdominal muscles in front, which pull up the pelvis, and the buttock muscles behind, which pull it down, thus rolling back the pelvis and flattening the hollow in the lumbar spine.

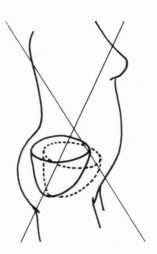

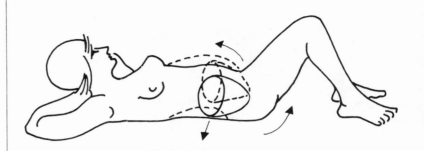

The pelvic basin and its contents must not tilt forward.

Pelvic tilting in its most elaborate form is exhibited in belly dancing, where the movements are from side-to-side as well as front-to-back. Most women usually perform similar motions during sexual intercourse; nevertheless this exercise is sometimes a little difficult to understand at first. Lying on the back with the knees bent is the easiest starting position for learning the basic front-to-back action which is important in the childbearing year. In late pregnancy, however, the weight of the uterus compresses the major blood vessels in this position, so if you experience discomfort or feel faint, practice this in one of the other recommended positions.

An analogy may help to make this clearer. In a sitting or standing position, think of your pelvis as a basin; place your hands on the bony crests at each hip — this is part of the upper rim. Just as you would tip back a basin to prevent the contents from spilling, so you tilt back your pelvis. Placing your hand in the hollow of your back may guide you also; you should feel the movement as the pelvis tilts backward.

Position: Lying on the back with knees bent.

Action: Roll the pelvis back by flattening the lower back down on the floor. Then make an extra effort. Contract the abdominal muscles on outward breath and tighten the buttock

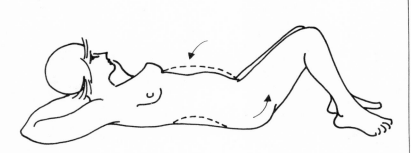

Active pelvic-tilting strengthens the abdominals and flattens the lower back.

muscles, too. Additional strong contraction of the muscles is necessary to make this an active strengthening exercise, not just a semipassive movement. To encourage more action in the lower abdominal muscles, place a hand just above the pubic bones so you can feel the muscles working. Hold the position for 3 seconds and then relax. Keep breathing!

Make sure that you do not raise your buttocks at all or shift your shoulders. Do not rock the pelvis upward as this will force the curve in the lower back. *Always emphasize the flattening of the hollow* and add as much additional abdominal wall retraction as you can. Postpartum, think about "making yourself thin" from front to back.

The pelvic floor can also be exercised at the same time.

The back-lying position is the easiest when you are first learning the exercise. The shoulders and hips are stabilized and gravity assists the backward tilt of the pelvis.

Progression: As pregnancy advances you have to control the pelvic tilt against the increasing weight of the pelvic contents. When you feel that you understand the correct movement, try it in the following positions as well.

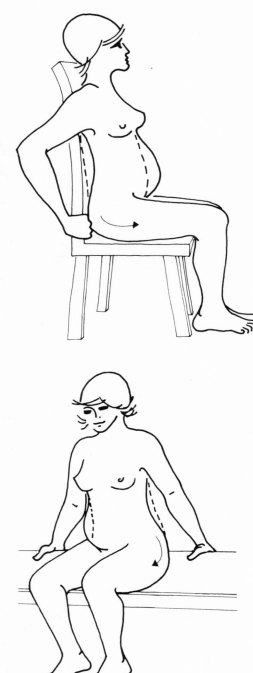

Side-lying

It is easier with knees bent — more movement can be felt — than with legs outstretched. The side-lying position is easier than three-fourths over (see page 99) when the pelvis is tilted unevenly.

A pillow between the legs can be used for comfort.

Sitting

This exercise is especially useful when seated in uncomfortable chairs or car seats, or on a waiting room bench. Reaching behind with your hands to grasp the back of the seat may help you to localize the action to the lumbar region.

Standing

See page 84. It takes practice to learn to do pelvic-tilting correctly, without moving other parts of the body, but this is essential for good posture. Check the side view in a mirror. Take care that you don't sway your upper trunk, and keep your legs still, with knees slightly bent, shoulders in neutral position, and arms held with palms forward.

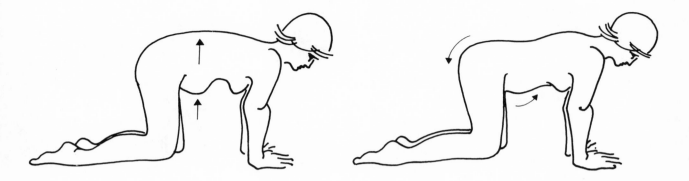

Pull up the pelvis and make a cat-back.   **Relax only to neutral.**

All-Fours

Pelvic-tilting on your hands and knees works the abdominal muscles against gravity. By having the shoulders and knees stabilized, you won't be tempted to move here, as you may be in the standing position and the action will be localized to the backbone. This exercise is sometimes called the cat-back or the "angry cat".

Until you get the feel of it, it is helpful to have somebody supervise you. It is difficult to tell at first whether the back is held at neutral, which it should be, or is hollowing, which is the opposite of what this exercise is intended to achieve. The force of gravity tends to make the back sag, and so does the weight of the uterus pulling down in pregnancy. Your partner can help by placing a hand over the *small of your back*, providing light guiding resistance so that you raise your backbone from here, rather than higher up (although the spine does move as a whole, of course). Imagine there is a string attached to the last bone of your spine (coccyx) and that you are pulling it up and letting it out.

Position: Hands directly under shoulders, knees under hips. Back held in neutral position with the small of the back (lumbar curve) flattened, *not hollowed*. Keep head aligned with the straight back.
     Keep elbows and knees still.

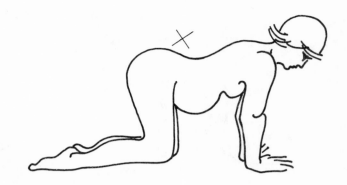

Never let the spine sag.

Action: Pull in your abdominal muscles and buttocks and press
    up with the lower back. Hold for a few seconds — then re-
    lax a little so that the back returns to *neutral* only. This
    means that you will still be holding the muscles a little
    tense to maintain this antigravity position. If you were to
    let go, as in other exercises, the lumbar spine would sink
    down into a curve; this must be avoided since the back
    muscles may go into spasm trying to counteract the drag of
    the weight underneath if the abdominal muscles are weak.

During the child-bearing year the essential focus of this
activity is to correct the pelvic tilt against the force of gravity.
Sometimes this exercise is expanded, in yoga for example, to
involve mobilization of the entire spine, "hollowing and hump-
ing" with the neck flexing and extending as well. However,
for our purposes it is important not to lose the key action amidst
extra movement. Furthermore, excessive mobilization of the
spinal joints and ligaments is not necessary through the maternity cycle as mobility has been achieved by the hormonal adjustments.

The all-fours position for the pelvic-tilting exercise and for
washing the floor or picking up things can improve comfort in
pregnancy (as long as the back doesn't hollow, which will cause
discomfort and the abdomen to sag). Removing the load of the
uterus off the backbone and out of the pelvis, where it presses
on the major blood vessels, for a while relieves circulation congestion, nerve twinges, and pelvic pressure. The baby often

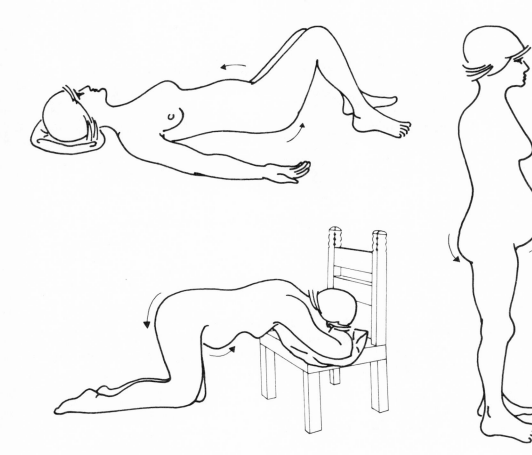

Pelvic-tilting can be done in many positions.

decides to adjust position, too, which may bring extra relief in pregnancy and labor. Going on hands and knees during transition has helped alleviate severe backache in labor and can assist rotation of the baby's head when the presentation is posterior. (The bony back of the baby's head, instead of the soft face, lies against the back of the mother's pelvis.)

Postpartum pelvic-tilting is highly motivating because your slack abdominals really droop when you're on all fours! (Again it is emphasized that this is *not* a mobility exercise for the spine but must be done slowly with *holding* to strengthen the muscles.)

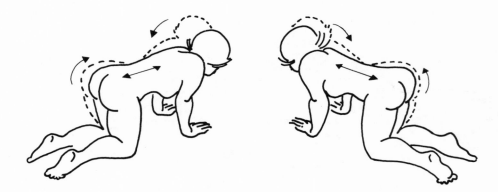

Bend from side to side without a hollow in the spine.

Side-Bending on All Fours

Also known as "tail-wagging," this exercise is a variation of all-fours and involves lateral or sideways tilting of the pelvis. The same position and principles apply: The aim is to maintain the condition of the abdominals and avoid excessive mobilization of the lumbar spine.

Action: With your back held at neutral, turn your head to the left, bending at the waist. Keep the back flat as you now turn back and bend your waist to the right.
This exercise uses both front and side abdominal muscles. The hollow in the back is corrected to neutral while the trunk flexes from side to side.

EXERCISE 3: LEG-SLIDING

Position: Lying on back, knees bent, pelvis tilted backward, and lumbar spine flattened. Keep breathing normally throughout.

Action: Hold the position of corrected pelvic tilt as, sliding the heels, you slowly stretch the legs out straight. If the abdominals are unable to keep the back flat, draw the knees back up again, one at a time, to the point where the spine began to arch. Work in this range until you can maintain a flattened back with the legs outstretched.

Progression: Leg-lowering with bent knees. See page 81.

Lowering the legs with bent knees, as described in this exercise, involves strong work from the lower half of the abdominal corset in order to hold the pelvis stable. It is always preferable to raising both legs with straight knees since you can control the descent of the legs within the limits of your muscle power. You start from the easiest part of the range, and when the weight of the legs and the force of gravity match your strength, you can bend the knees a little to reduce the leverage and ease the strain and allow the heels to rest on the floor. By stopping at this point you avoid losing control of the corrected pelvic tilt. Double-leg–raising (see page 17) is a movement that *begins* at the point of maximum difficulty and exertion. You will not know if you cannot hold your back flat until it *has* arched, as you strain to lift both legs off the ground simultaneously.

EXERCISE 4: STRAIGHT CURL-UP

Prenatal: This exercise is for early starters. If you are well into the last trimester and cannot readily perform these movements, then do not try. If the recti muscles have parted, from this pregnancy or a previous one, postpone this exercise and concentrate on supporting the muscles and raising just the head at first, as described on page 60.
Postpartum: Always check the midline of your abdominal wall before doing this exercise. If the recti muscles have separated, support them as described on page 62; this is actually a progression of the same exercise.

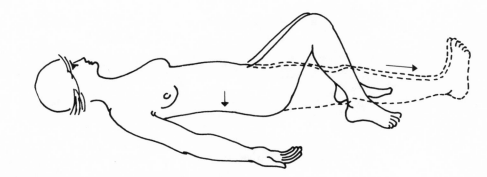

Flatten the lower back as you slowly slide the heels down.

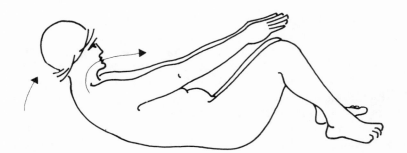

Curl up just halfway to the knees.

Position: Lying on the back with knees bent, pelvis tilted back.

Action: Bring your chin onto your chest. As you breathe out, fold forward without any jerking or hinging movement. Come up just as far as the back naturally bends with the waist still down on the surface. This is about 8 inches or an angle of 45°.

Slowly return to the starting position; don't drop back. The arms are held outstretched in front at first, to aid the trunk.

Progression: Arms can be folded in front, then clasped behind head. See page 80.

Self-test: If you cannot perform the basic straight curl-up, do the preliminary strengthening exercise.

Preliminary Strengthening Exercise (Straight Sit-Back)

Position: Sitting close to your bent knees.

Action: Stretch your arms out in front and lean backwards a little way; then sit forward again. You should have complete control of the position since you move up away from the strain as soon as the force of gravity matches your muscle strength.

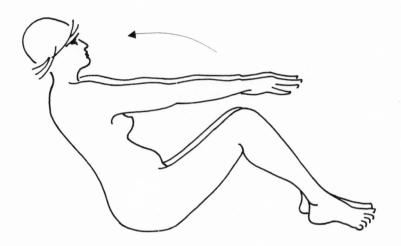

Increase the distance so that you gradually roll further back to the floor before moving up to your knees again.

Perform the movement with just the abdominal muscles, although you may rest your arms on your knees between sit-backs.

EXERCISE 5. DIAGONAL CURL-UP

If there is a separation of the recti muscles (see page 62), postpone this exercise until the condition has been corrected. *Prenatal:* This exercise is also for early starters, although it is a little easier than the straight curl-up since you move obliquely and have more help from other muscles in the corset. If you are in the last trimester and cannot perform this movement with ease and comfort, then do not try.

Position: Lying on the back with knees bent.

Action: Bring your chin onto your chest. As you breathe out, fold forward reaching with your outstretched arms to the outside of the left knee. Slowly return back to the starting position. Repeat the movement to the right knee.

Progression: Arms can be folded across the chest, or clasped behind the neck, see page 80.

Self-test: If you cannot perform the basic diagonal curl-up, do the preliminary strengthening exercise.

Move diagonally with outstretched arms to the opposite knee: to the left and back . . . to the right and back.

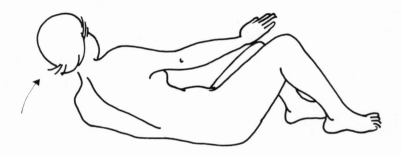

Preliminary Strengthening Exercise (Diagonal Sit-Back)

Position: Sitting close to your bent knees.

Action: Stretch your arms out to the side of the left knee and lean back a little. As you come forward again, direct your arms to the outside of the right knee. You should have complete control of the position since you move up into the easier part of the range as soon as you feel any strain.

    The abdominal muscles alone should perform the movement, but you can rest your arms on your knees between times. Remember to keep your back rounded.

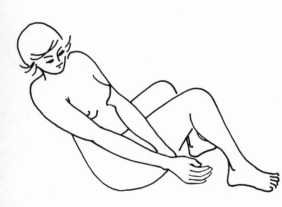

Progressive Abdominal Exercises for Early Pregnancy and Later Postpartum

Prenatal: Exercises should be commenced as soon as possible, preferably before pregnancy! But these stronger exercises should not be begun after obvious changes occur in pregnancy, when the abdomen becomes prominent and the abdominal corset has expanded. The enlarging abdomen alters the angle at which the muscles, particularly the recti, exert their force; they must shorten over a progressively larger curve. The increased weight of the trunk may tempt you to stabilize your feet, but remember that this will encourage the hip flexors to pull more strongly on the spine with its softened ligaments and against the diminishing power of the stretched abdominal muscles.

Postpartum: When you feel stronger and can easily perform the essential exercises, they can be progressed. After the muscles have regained their shape and elasticity, you need to demand more work of them so that strength is built up.

Trained supervision is rarely available, which is why this book aims to help you understand the principles so you can be your own guide. The exercises can be modified according to your individual level of tolerance, prior training, labor and delivery experience, and postpartum management. You should also engage regularly in some aerobic activity that provides basic fitness, but the abdominal muscles, like those of the pelvic floor, require special attention — particularly during the childbearing year.

1. *The position of the arms:* Curl-ups can be made more difficult by altering the position of the arms so that the leverage is increased. The easiest way is to use them to help you move forward, stretching them out in front as was done in exercises number 4 and 5. It is harder when the arms are folded on your chest and not helping you to curl forward. *Normal strength* is present when you can execute a smooth curl-up and roll-back with the hands clasped behind your head. Now the arms have been used to make the lever longer. This can be further progressed with arms held above your head, or even holding a weight. The arms must stay above your head and must not be used to provide momentum.

2. *The position of the legs:* When the legs are used to add leverage, the lower abdominals work strongly as the legs are lowered and straightened in one coordinated movement. The knees can be further flexed or the heels rested down at any time to prevent strain. Do not straighten the legs before you start to lower them as this greater leverage makes the pelvic tilt too difficult to control. *Normal strength* has been achieved when you are able to hold the legs straight at an angle of 45° for a few seconds. Do

not try to lower the legs below this angle or you will get into the "seesaw" problems described in double-leg–raising (p. 17) and the lower back will arch as the pelvic tilt is lost. Instead, you can progress the exercise by holding the position longer (keep breathing!) or spreading and closing the legs at this angle. Legs can be raised from a sitting position for greater resistance from gravity; the abdominals work hard to stabilize the pelvic tilt. (The V-Sit is an example, where you balance on your seat with both arms and legs outstretched. The leverage and effects of gravity demand maximum power to hold this position.)

3. *The position of the trunk:* It has been seen that less muscle work is required for trunk movements in the middle range where the force of gravity is also reduced. The closer your head is to the horizontal level, the stronger the muscle contraction required to raise you forward, and more so if the trunk must come up from a slant board or other downward-inclining surface.

Folding the arms across the chest is a way to progress the curl-ups.

Hands behind the head is the most challenging position for curl-ups.

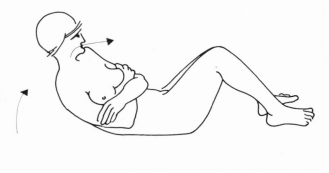

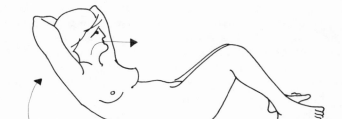

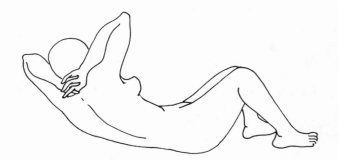

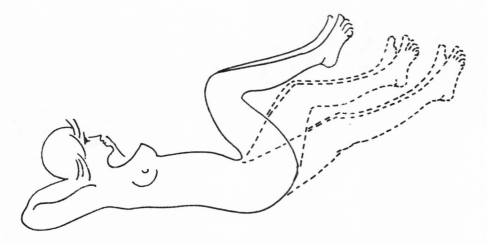

Keep the lower back flat as you lower and straighten your legs.

4. *The number of repetitions:* In the past, exercise programs were popular that provided for an ever-increasing number of repetitions, as well as a decrease in the resting interval between them. Relaxation — the equally significant component of muscle activity — was thus neglected, and it has been found that multirepetitions tend to produce stiffness and fatigue. A specific exercise need not be performed more than 5 times in sequence, although the program can be repeated later. You can also interchange exercises so that you come back to certain muscle groups that need extra attention. As you improve in strength, it is more encouraging to progress the position or the leverage rather than perform tiresome repetitions. Intervals of rest and correct breathing are as important as the exercise itself. Always do the exercise slowly enough for it to be executed completely and for you to retain control of the position and movement at all times.

Posture and Comfort 4

POSTURE HAS TO DO with looking well and feeling well —
whether you are male, female, young, old, pregnant, or postpartum. If you feel down in the dumps, your negative emotional state will be registered in a slumped, droopy posture. If
you feel great, you'll stand tall and walk with a spring in your
step. This is just basic body language. Since posture is so
influenced by one's feelings, during pregnancy you really need
to learn how to carry your body and baby best so that you don't
feel awkward, clumsy, or misshapen. Naturally posture varies
with different body types but there are certain guidelines that
determine good alignment and enhance balance and muscle
action.

Your posture may have been faulty before you became pregnant, but fortunately, since feeling and habits play such a de-
termining role, it is usually correctable. In some cases, considerable muscle and ligament adaptation has occurred and the
process of re-education requires more effort. Basically what you
have to achieve is efficiency and endurance — that is, minimal
effort and fatigue — in all your resting and working positions.
This efficiency is gained by good body alignment, which results from adequate supports and easy coordination of the various body segments. Unnecessary tension and stress on muscles
and ligaments and cramping of pelvic and abdominal organs
are avoided.

Posture, as we learned in Chapter 1, is controlled by postural reflexes, by which the brain communicates with certain
signal stations in the body — the ears, eyes, and muscles being
the most important. We can see the nature of this reflex by
watching the uncoordinated actions of someone who is blind-
folded. Because the reflex occurs, as the term indicates, at an
automatic level, we are often unaware of bad habits we may
have developed. Attention to a few details while you are pregnant can increase your comfort enormously and help you to
cultivate good posture during changing bodily states. Postpartum, when the extra weight has gone, it is important that

you readjust and do not continue the stance that you developed in pregnancy. Whereas during pregnancy the changes were gradual, after delivery you will have to adapt quickly and must at first consciously brace the stretched supporting muscles, namely, the abdominals and the pelvic floor.

Posture involves adjustments to the force of gravity, which is why reclining is more restful than being upright. Postural defects are seen most clearly in the standing position, where the body segments are aligned to maintain a state of muscular equilibrium around the line of gravity. Once humans stood up on two legs, the vertebral column became subject to compression; the natural curves formed in the spine are a compromise between flexibility and stability. In pregnancy they become accentuated as the center of gravity moves forward. Since this shift in the center of gravity increases the load on the spine, the woman tends to stand further back on her heels. Further compensation may occur such as bringing the head and shoulders forward, increasing the lumbar curve, or swaying back from the waist. Backache commonly results from this incorrect weight distribution since the muscles of the back are doing extra work.

Something that frequently affects posture — along with emotions, habits, muscle power, and ligaments — is *shoes*. Comfortable and supportive shoes aid both your disposition and your appearance! High heels throw your pelvis and body weight forward, which hollows the back and strains ligaments in the hips and knees. Because of this unstable position the muscles have to work much harder, and the weight on your toes may cause the arches and balls of the feet to protest. If you are accustomed to wearing high heels, it will be hard to adjust to low heels or flats because your calf muscles will have shortened and they need time to stretch gradually. Shoes with a minus heel stretch these muscles even more than flats and may be uncomfortable to wear at first. However, many women find them comfortable if they have worn these shoes from the beginning of pregnancy, before the weight shifts back toward the feet. If you first try wearing these shoes after the sixth month, your postural muscles will be hard-pressed to compensate doubly for the forward shift in the center of gravity *and* the minus heel. While it is great to walk barefoot in sand, the usual hard surface beneath us needs a buffer. The sole of the shoe should be thick and resilient and the shoe's shank underneath the inner arch should provide support when you stand. If you can press the arch down just with your hand, it is inadequate, and an extra arch support may be necessary as you gain weight during the pregnancy. Painful pressure under the ball of the foot can be relieved by a metatarsal footpad, available in drugstores. The ideal shoe does not change the shape of your foot in any way; the toes are not squeezed and the heel should fit firmly, slanting neither to one side nor the other.

Posture in Standing

This is ideally an ongoing process, not an occasional exercise. You may have been told many times in your life to stand up straight for esthetic reasons, but in pregnancy you need to do so for physiological reasons. Research has shown that ligaments play the major role when standing at ease. But during the childbearing year the supporting muscles must do their share so that you don't rely on the softened ligaments to withstand the stresses of pregnancy. The spinal column forms a subtle s-curve around the line of gravity; the more pronounced the curve, the more muscle work is demanded. The position of the pelvis, which supports the spinal column, is always important and in pregnancy you have to develop a keener sense of the pelvic tilt. This pelvic angle determines the prominence of both your abdomen and bottom and is significant for appearance as well as comfort. Naturally the pelvis tends to angle forward because of the increasing weight of its contents and the stretching of the abdominal wall. You need to make a special effort to keep the pelvis tilted backward — pulling it up at the front with the abdominal muscles and down at the back with the buttock muscles. It is exactly the action described on pages 67–68, which can be done in many positions. In standing, it is most difficult to do correctly because there may be, without your knowing it, compensation from knee or shoulder movements. Placing one hand on the abdomen and the other under the buttocks helps to guide the right movement. If prolonged forward tilt of the pelvis is allowed, the muscles in front will weaken, the muscles behind will shorten, and consequently the curve in the lower back will be increased. The fulcrum for all these forces of stress is the point at which the spinal column joins the pelvis, the commonest region of backache. See page 8 for the drawing of this bowstring effect.

The position of the head is significant in influencing the state of the rest of the body. If you let your head slump and look at the ground, the body will droop. Just drawing up the back of the neck and tucking the chin in above the notch between the collarbones helps to bring all the body segments into line. Think ''tall'' and hold your head high, as if an invisible thread were pulling up from your head to the ceiling. Shoulders and hips should be level; if you wear a belt it should be parallel to the ground. Since in pregnancy it makes no sense to think about pulling in your belly, concentrate on tucking under your bottom. Postpartum, you need to watch the pelvic tilt carefully as well, consciously bracing the abdominal and buttock muscles at first until they are strong enough to control the lumbar curve.

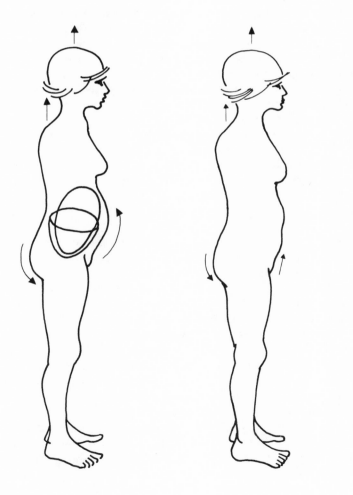

Observe the different features of the two postures shown in the drawing on page 163. Stand comfortably and ask a friend whether you exhibit any of the key postural defects: chin poked forward, shoulders rounded, pelvis tilted to the front, one or both legs pressed back or feet turned in or out. Women often stand with one hip slouched, too, possibly a habit developed in adolescence when girls are frequently taller than boys and self-consciously try to appear shorter. You can check yourself now and then in front of mirrors and store windows, but remember that it is the side view that is most revealing.

Practice holding the corrected position and then relaxing — which probably means that you will slump back to your old faulty position! As you practice relaxing and correcting, you will develop the sensation of good posture because your muscles will learn to send in new messages. Don't ever exaggerate by throwing the shoulders back, which hollows the lumbar spine, or pulling the elbows too far back so that the head and shoulders move forward. Postural exercises require that you develop a sense of what *feels* correct. So perform them slowly and hold for about 10 seconds before relaxing. Relaxation is also a component of muscle action and should never be neglected, or muscles become tense and tight. Standing with the eyes closed heightens postural awareness, improves balance, and surprisingly is a relaxation experience.

Progressions in Standing

Stand, back to wall, but with your feet a few inches away from it, arms at side, palms facing forward. Make contact with the head, shoulders, and buttocks. Press back the shoulders and trunk but not the knees, and try to flatten the curves in the neck and lower back. Next, raise the arms sideways while keeping them in contact with the wall at all times. Then bring arms upward to the ears, back to shoulder level, and finally down again. Holding these positions against the wall will help you increase the endurance of the muscles that maintain the body in correct alignment. Also this corrective stretching of tired or tight muscles feels terrific and relieves backache. During tedious desk or household jobs, riding in an elevator or standing in line near a wall, it's a good idea to "iron out" and relax the ache or stiffness in the back from time to time. Do not try to walk away from the wall while holding the body braced. You will look like a tin soldier and may become dependent on the wall for your starting position! Besides, you assume a multitude of different postures throughout the day and as your muscles get into good shape and your awareness of them improves, you will demonstrate better posture.

Standing still for long periods of time is very tiring; the muscles work statically to hold the body position stable against the push of gravity but the uncomfortable strain develops foremost as a result of circulatory effects. Half of the blood volume is below heart level in the upright position and movement provides relief by allowing the muscles to rest and work alternately, which keeps the circulation moving, and this is particularly important in pregnancy as the blood volume is increased. As much as you can, avoid prolonged standing, since the blood must take an uphill path back to the heart unaided by the pumping of the muscles. If you do have to wait for public transport or if you work standing without a seat, there are a few things you can do to keep the muscles active. Shift your weight from one foot to the other — side to side or diagonally back and forth; go up on your toes and back on the heels (resting your hand on some firm support for balance). Press your toes into your shoes and try to raise the arches of the feet. Blood is returned from the legs to the heart by a "venous pump," which is muscle action in the legs, because veins, unlike arteries, do not have muscular walls to maintain pressure. Valves placed in the thin-walled veins direct the blood; if they are forced to support a back-up of blood flow, the veins become distended. If there is too much pooling of venous blood in the legs, you will feel faint. This is the body's way of protecting itself; when no muscular contractions are pumping the blood back uphill to the heart, and blood pressure falls, you feel the need to recline or may be forced eventually to fall to the ground. Then the blood can be returned to the heart more easily.

Because the venous blood must be returned against the force of gravity when the body is upright, and since the increased blood volume and growing pressure within the abdomen tax the circulatory system in pregnancy, the veins may become more prominent and perhaps varicosed. Exercise and frequent change of position also relieves pain in the groin. This may be felt in late pregnancy when the mother is standing and results from spasm of the muscle fibers in the round ligament of the uterus. These painful twinges, and the pressure and discomfort felt in the groin, can be relieved by your partner raising and lowering your hips while you are lying down. This activity is similar to lifting a wheelbarrow. You relax completely with your legs loose and bent so that the thighs can be grasped.

Relief is usually immediate after the uterus has been tipped back a few times off the cramped structures. Excessive sitting should also be avoided during pregnancy since this compounds pelvic pressure and congestion.

Especially in pregnancy, no one position is comfortable for long. On the following pages we will consider various positions and how they can be used more effectively to increase comfort and improve body function. The sense of poise and well-being achieved with good posture makes these small efforts worthwhile. In pregnancy and postpartum, you look as well as you feel. Sometimes trying to look better makes you feel better.

Posture in Sitting

Posture and comfort in sitting are important since this position is the one most frequently used. The chair seat should

Good posture in sitting

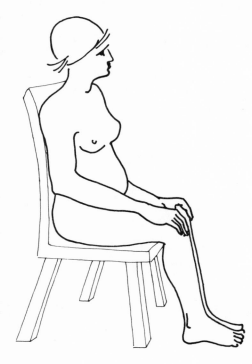

Comfort is increased with pillows and a footrest.

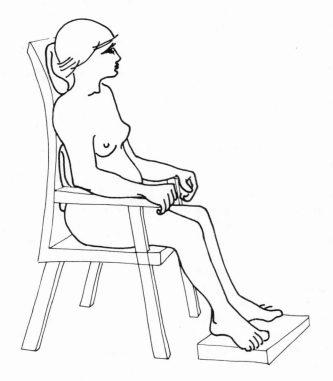

support the length of the thigh. It should be high enough from the ground so your knee is not forced into a higher position than your hips (in pregnancy the muscles in front of the hip joints tend to become tight). During pregnancy, the legs are most comfortable when spread apart to prevent compression on the abdomen, with your feet not tucked underneath you but supported on the floor, or a stool, out in front of you. Make sure that the lumbar spine is supported. You may need to place a little cushion in the small of your back because the design of many chairs and car seats is deficient here. (Don't create a larger curve with a large, unyielding pillow!) Chairs with high backs to support the head and shoulders are ideal for practicing relaxation, especially since we spend so much time sitting. Another cushion at the back of the neck may increase comfort. Take every opportunity to elevate the feet, preferably with calves supported, when you are sitting. This is also a good opportunity to do foot-stretching and -rotating exercises, which will aid the circulation from the legs (see pages 118–119), relieving

Elevate and rotate the feet when resting.

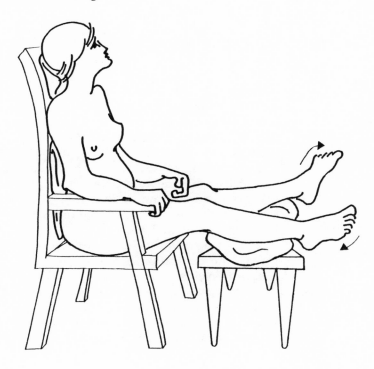

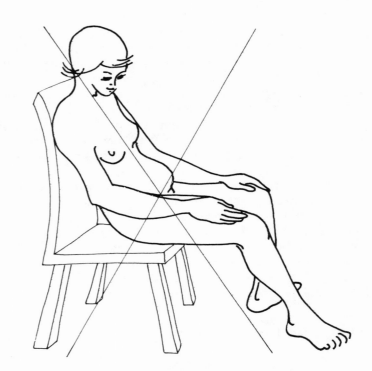

Don't slump on the edge of a chair like this!

congestion and ache from varicose veins if they are present. When your feet rest on the floor, "walk" them up and down from the toes. Don't just sit on the edge of a chair — use the back support to keep from slumping forward with rounded shoulders. In pregnancy, this pressure and restriction on the abdomen can cause indigestion. When you stand up again, use your legs to raise your body; don't pull on adjacent furniture. It's worth investing in a high stool so that you can take the weight off your feet when you're working at high surfaces, the ironing board, and so on.

Sitting with knees crossed causes pressure that interferes with the circulation of the blood, which, in turn, can cause varicose veins. This position should be avoided, especially during pregnancy. The position also tightens the very hip muscles that you want to be stretched and limbered during pregnancy.

While sitting at a desk, rest your head on your hands occasionally to relieve tension in the neck and shoulders. In pregnancy, spread the legs apart and allow the abdomen to relax forward. If you're typing, make sure that you are seated high enough to avoid pain between the shoulder blades from excess muscle holding while your hands work.

When feeding your baby, do not sit with rounded shoulders and lean over the child. Instead, support the baby and your arm on a pillow, or raise your thigh by putting your foot on a stool or the rung of a chair. This way you can keep your

Perch on a stool when working at high surfaces.

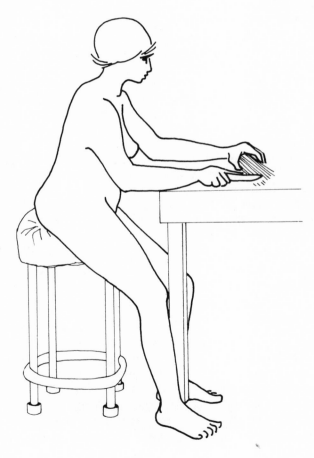

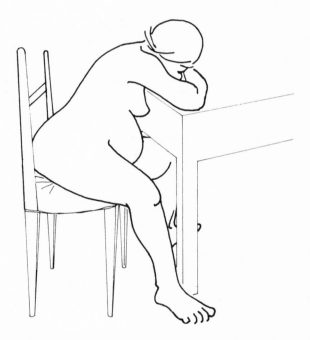

Rest like this occasionally when at a desk or table.

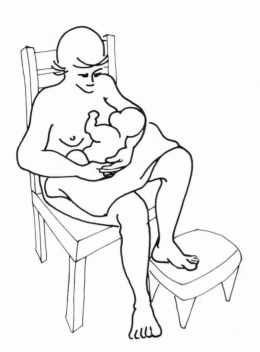

Sit with maximum support and comfort for feeding baby.

back straight, resting against the chair. Since feeding is one of your main activities postpartum, these little details do make a difference in preventing discomfort in the shoulder region. Shoulder-rotating exercises (pages 101–102) are recommended to relieve upper backache if it develops during feeding sessions.

Sitting in the car: If you drive a sporty model and the bucket seats are uncomfortably low, try sitting on a cushion so that your knees are level with your hips. Support for the lower back is often necessary, especially during long drives, which also cause the accumulation of considerable muscle tension for the driver. The neck, shoulder blades, and right leg are affected, along with the lower back. Frequent breaks help allay fatigue and discomfort for both the driver and passenger.

Many women feel that they should not wear seatbelts during pregnancy. On the contrary, research on expectant mothers who were involved in automobile accidents reveals that belts should be worn. The two-section strap has been shown to be the most effective and both the shoulder restraint and the lower strap should be as taut as possible (if they are adjustable). The abdominal strap should be below the bulge, and a small cushion between you and the strap may make you more comfortable. This cushion also provides more protection for the baby, who is floating in a fluid environment and is therefore less restrained.

An infant car seat is necessary for your new baby's safety. *Purchase one now.* Carrying your newborn home from the hospital in your arms is just not safe. Consumer organizations and the American Academy of Pediatricians review and make recommendations from the brands available on the market. Some seats are convertible to other uses.

Posture in Lying

Prone (lying on your front)

It is usually with regret that women have to give up lying comfortably on their abdomens as their pregnancies advance. Then, because one sits or lies mostly with hips and knees bent, the muscles in front of the hip joints may become shortened, which makes achieving and maintaining good posture a little difficult. So do try to rest and sleep in the prone position for as long as you can, using pillows for comfort as needed. However, don't

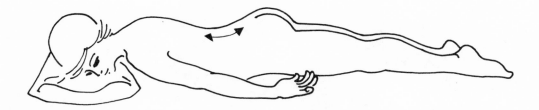

Lying prone without a pillow under the hips: note sag in mattress permitting the back to hollow.

pile several under your chin or you will force your back into the uncomfortable lumbar strain that this position is designed to avoid and you will cause faulty placement of head and shoulders. If you have been accustomed to this, it will take time to decrease gradually the number of pillows. Postpartum, most mothers are very glad to be able to enjoy this position again; others may need reminding and a few may feel it is an effort to adjust the bed and roll over! But there are many benefits of lying on your front after delivery, and these should give the position high priority with you:

- It feels fantastic!
- Your stitches won't bother you. So it's an excellent position for practicing pelvic floor contractions and pelvic tilting.
- Back strain is relieved; the abdominal wall is relaxed . . . if you have a pillow under your hips. And you must place a pillow there to achieve the correct pelvic tilt, or you will sink a little into the mattress, actually forming that unde-

Lying prone with a pillow under the hips: note the raised pelvis, flattened back, and relaxed abdominals.

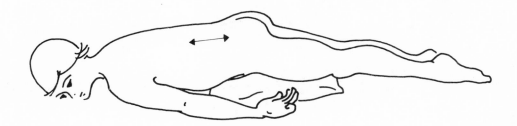

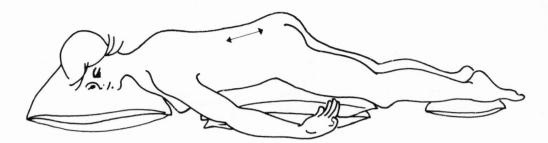

Extra pillows relieve pressure on the breasts: two at the hips and one at the chest keep the pelvic tilt correct.

sirable hollow back. Prolonged prone lying without suitable support, especially if you prop on your elbows to read or chat, can strain the back ligaments. Lying on your front is a resting or sleeping position.

- It helps to tip the uterus forward when the latter returns within the pelvis, without the risks of the knee-chest position, which was used in former times. Anyway, the importance of the position of the uterus is debatable these days. Other pelvic organs are also encouraged to resume their normal places.

Rest in this position at least twice a day for an hour or so. You may even wish to sleep prone. If at any time your breasts are too sore to lie on, try putting two pillows under your hips and one beneath your chin and shoulders. That way no pressure is

Never lie prone like this postpartum!

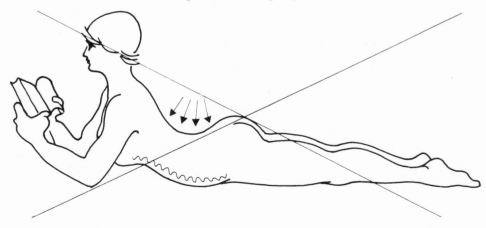

put on your breasts and you maintain the proper angle of flat back with relaxed abdominal muscles. Note in the drawing that the pillow(s) is placed under the hips — *not* under the central abdomen. If it is too high you'll soon feel discomfort in your stomach and your back, which will be strained. Place the pillow a little lower till you feel the pelvis tilted in a comfortable position. If it doesn't feel good, then you haven't got the pillow quite right. The pillow is important since mattresses are rarely as firm as they really should be.

Supine (lying on your back)

In pregnancy, as the weight of the uterus increases, compression of the major veins in the abdomen can occur when you are in the supine position, and this can result in low blood pressure. If lying on your back makes you feel faint or in any other way uncomfortable, then avoid this position as much as possible. In labor, this is a particularly undesirable position; contractions may be diminished and the baby's heart rate (which normally drops during a contraction) may be further reduced if "supine hypotension," or low blood pressure, results from compression of major blood vessels by the uterus. Furthermore, many women suffer backache in labor and feel more comfortable in other positions. Research indicates that supine is the least favorable (although the most widespread) position for enhancing the progress of labor.

Many women, however, prefer to lie on their backs, and they experience no adverse symptoms. There will be many occasions when you will be asked to lie supine: for checks and examinations during labor; for allowing the fetal heart monitor, if it is used, to be applied to your abdominal wall; for learning

Comfort in the supine position

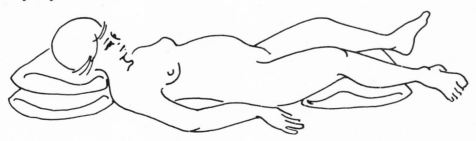

some of the prenatal exercises; and so on. In several of these cases you can modify the position to elevate your back and relax the legs. The following suggestions should make you more comfortable:

- *A folded towel* or *small* cushion provides support to the small of the back if the surface is either too hard or too soft. (A regular pillow is too large).
- *Bending the knees,* or relaxing them over a pillow, will take the traction off the abdomen and flatten the hollow in the back. If you plan to sleep this way, make sure the pillow is under the thighs. This will flex and relax the joints but will not cut off circulation, as might a pillow pressing into the back of the knees. Flat on back, legs outstretched is not a recommended position for comfort in later pregnancy!
- You may care to take a rest in the back-lying position and *elevate your feet.* This will aid circulation in the legs, and help ease varicose veins, cramps, and the like. The foot of your bed can be slightly raised if you suffer from constant aching in the legs, and this is often recommended as a routine measure to aid venous return overnight which occurs in whatever position you lie. In order to aid the return of blood from the veins in the legs, you need to elevate the feet only so they are *just higher than your heart.*

Take every opportunity to elevate your feet.

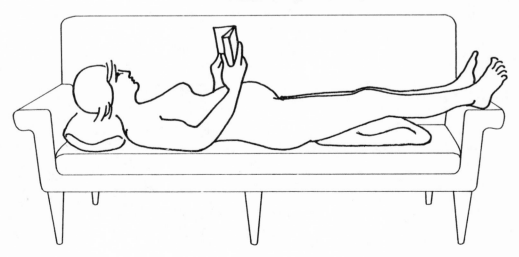

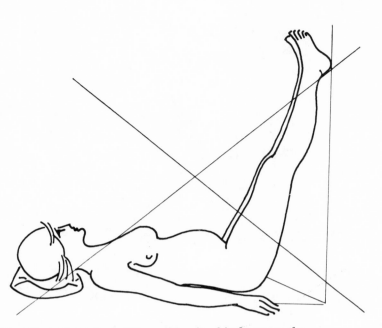

The effect of gravity in this position is a hindrance to the circulation, not a help!

In fact, if you raise the legs to near-vertical heights you actually hinder the circulation. The major veins returning blood from the legs can be compressed in the groin, and the effect of gravity in this position causes the valves in the veins to collapse, resulting in the pooling of blood. Resting with the length of your legs against the wall, therefore, is unnecessary and will actually worsen the condition you are trying to relieve. It is also rather difficult to maneuver oneself in and out of this position and it is potentially harmful if you suddenly lose your balance. Walking, however, is superior to passive resting positions in affecting the return of blood to the heart.

Posture in Half-Lying

This is the position you probably assume when reading in bed, and it is the one in which you will spend most of the immediate days postpartum. Usually the knees are a little bent and the legs roll out comfortably from the hips. However, there can be a problem with the lower back. If you lie for prolonged periods without support in the lumbar area, ligaments can be stretched,

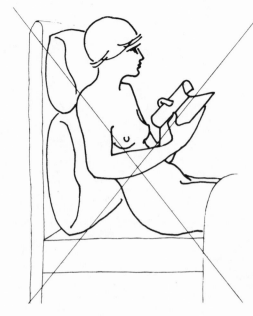

Don't slouch when half-lying.

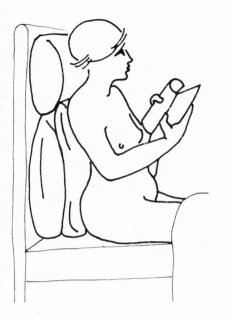

Use pillows to support your spine.

giving rise to joint instability and pain. There are long liga-ments at both the front and back of the spine which can be strained at either extreme — when the backbone is excessively hollowed *or* rounded. One orthopedic specialist calls this the "nursing mother's position," but it is easy for all of us to slouch in the bed like this. An extra pillow makes all the difference, as you see.

Posture in Side-Lying

Most women in pregnancy and labor probably achieve the greatest comfort from lying on their sides. The abdominal weight is eased off the lower back and groin, compression of major blood vessels is avoided, and the joints are loosely flexed. Occasionally strain may be felt in the uppermost hip, but this can be prevented by placing a pillow *lengthwise* between the legs. Make sure your upper foot is also resting on the pillow for better relaxation; if it is just hanging it will be doing muscle work in response to gravity. The edge of a pillow or a rolled towel tucked underneath the abdomen can relieve any strain on

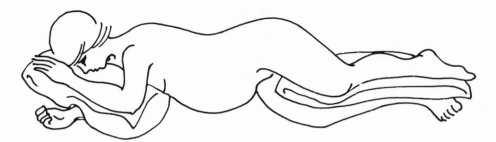

Comfort in side-lying—note pillow between the legs.

the lower back that may arise. It is easier to turn from this position onto the back for examinations during labor compared to the position that will be described next. Also, when you are lying directly on your side rather than three-quarters over during contractions, the uterus has more freedom to tip forward.

Posture in Three-Quarters Over

Here you lie more toward the front than you do in the side-lying position. You may prefer to have the underneath arm behind your back; this will bring your shoulders further over. The pillow under your head can also be used to rest your upper-

Comfort when lying three-quarter over supported by pillows.

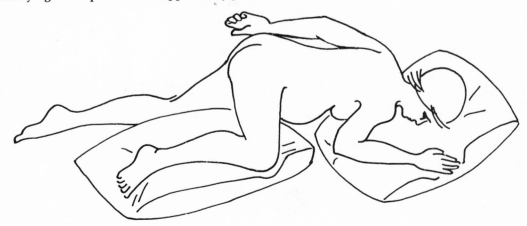

most arm. A second pillow can support the front leg for increased comfort. This position is a favorite for resting and sleeping during pregnancy. In labor, however, the side-lying position is preferable because it prevents your putting your body weight on the uterus as it contracts.

Posture on All Fours

The all-fours position, described on pages 71–73, exercises the abdominal wall against gravity (you must not let your back sag!) and relieves backache and pelvic pressure. Circulation is also aided by a change to this position since the compression of the uterus is temporarily removed from the back and the pelvic floor. This can relieve cramps in the thighs, buttocks, or groin, and can ease the discomfort of hemorrhoids and vaginal swelling, which are symptoms of pelvic pressure and congestion. This position can also help backache or tired legs that come from continual standing. Take any opportunity, when doing things at floor level, to get down on your hands and knees so that you can obtain these benefits. This position, or a modification of it when you kneel with elbows supported, is often used for comfort during labor and delivery.

Posture in Tailor-Sitting

It's too bad that we take chairs so much for granted and don't sit like this more often! In this position the lower back is nicely rounded — in fact, you need to take care not to slouch and particularly not to "lean" on the uterus.

A considerable number of women find that when their ankles are crossed their knees are a long way from the ground. Others will be so limber that they can place the soles of their feet together and still have their thighs in contact with the floor. Remember that people always show anatomical variation and difference in the tightness of ligaments, so the joints must never be forced. (*Warning:* Do not do these hip exercises if you experience any pain in the area of the pubic bones as separation at this fibrous union may be present.) Because women are taught from the time they are little girls to sit with their legs together or crossed, the muscles and ligaments of many women's inner thighs, especially the inward rotators of the hip, have usually shortened. It is quite a psychological as well as physical change

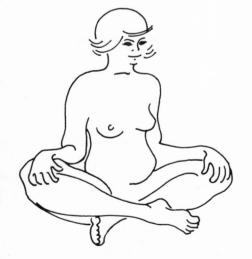

Sit like a tailor whenever you can.

to start to open up your legs and sit with them wide apart! (Stirrups, if you require them, are adjustable and in many cases avoidable if you prefer just to relax your legs on the bed, letting them flop to the side with the knees bent.) The psychological preparation may be even more important than the physical since women are so culturally unaccustomed to spreading their thighs like this. During delivery it is *essential* to relax the pelvic floor, so you need to feel at ease with your legs spread out.

Pushing your knees toward the floor is not recommended. Rather than increasing the range of movement, the body's most powerful reflex — the stretch reflex — will be invoked and cause these muscles to contract — *not* to relax or lengthen. You can increase the range more effectively by pressing both your knees toward the floor while providing resistance with your hands underneath the knees. Then as your thigh muscles — now a little tired — relax, your knees will drop farther apart. This activity also strengthens your pectoral muscles, which lie beneath the breasts. Don't bounce, but sustain the stretch.

You can also *work the outer thigh muscles actively* to bring the knees nearer to the floor, which, according to a law of physiology, relaxes the inner thighs.

While tailor-sitting, you will feel good if you stretch your arms and mobilize your shoulder region. Sometimes the shoulders drag forward and press on nerves, which can cause ting-

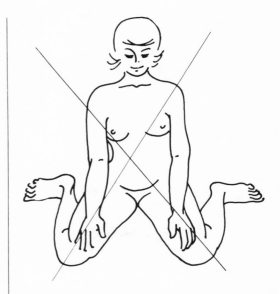

Avoid sitting in reverse-tailor fashion which strains the pubic area, knees and feet.

Exercise your outer thigh muscles to bring the knees closer to the floor.

Resist the downward movement of the knees to gain relaxation of the inner thigh muscles.

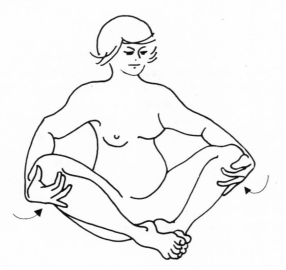

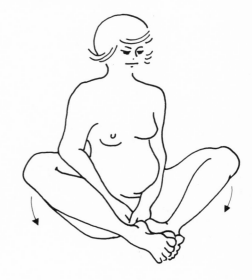

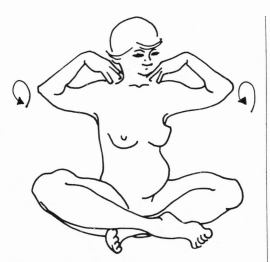

Shoulder-rotating relieves upper backache from poor posture or heavy breasts.

Stretch the arms — first right, then left. This relieves pressure under the ribs.

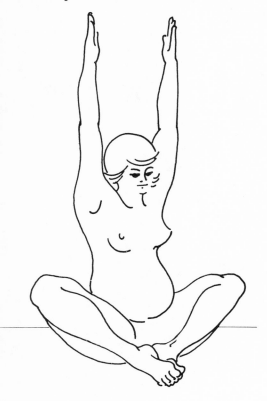

ling or numbness in the fingertips. Placing fingers on each shoulder and making circles *backward* with the elbows can relieve these symptoms and relieve upper backache from the weight of the breasts and feeding sessions. Stretching the arms over your head — reaching higher with the right, then higher with the left, and so forth — smooths out tightness in the shoulders and upper back and relieves the pressure under the rib cage in later pregnancy that gives rise to heartburn, breathlessness, and discomfort. An added lift is gained if you bend to the opposite side while stretching. Don't arch the lower back at all during these movements; you can try them leaning against the wall.

Long-sitting on the bed or floor with the legs straight out and apart is another position you may like to try for a change when reading or watching TV. Foot-bending and stretching exercises can be done at the same time and these movements will help to stretch the calf muscles. In the long-sitting position, the lumbar spine is rounded but the hamstrings are on stretch — which you may feel if your knees don't rest flat on the floor as they should. Don't force them down; instead, gently bend and press your knees until the muscles are flexible enough to allow the joints to extend and, for most people, to touch the toes with the fingertips. Tight hamstrings increase the lumbar hollow so it is recommended that you practice sitting like this to lengthen them, easing out any stiffness in the lower back as you gently lean forward and back.

It is now well recognized that this safe way of actively stretching the hamstrings and the lower back is preferable to bending over in a standing position and forcefully trying to touch the floor. Attempting to keep the palms flat while the knees are "locked" back (also known as the monkey-walk position) is worse. It would also be hazardous were it not for the extreme difficulty in performing this strange feat and the sharp pain that is registered in the hamstring tendons, which fortunately serves as a warning sign! After touching the floor comes the task of raising the trunk upward against gravity, using the back muscles in their most inefficient role. In pregnancy this is even more undesirable because of the increased weight of the trunk, which the back muscles must lift, and the softening ligaments, which are vulnerable to strain. In any case, the back should never be worked in this way; instead, the legs must be used when the trunk is raised or lowered as we shall see in the section on body mechanics and lifting.

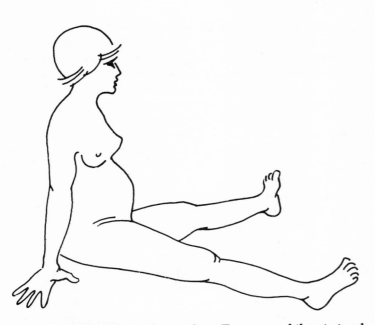

Support your back and stretch your legs. Try now and then to touch your toes, holding the stretch, not bouncing.

Exercises to strengthen the back muscles can be done in both tailor-sitting and long-sitting. Press the back against the wall and move both arms sideways and upward. Hold the position for a few seconds to get the feel of the straightened position which will help you to improve your posture. These muscles work against gravity to support the neck and upper trunk, for example, when inclined over a desk or table. Their weakness is commonly seen in round-shoulders, forward-poking head, and some degree of hunchback.

Always *relax* the muscles after holding the stretched position so that they don't become stiff.

Posture in Squatting

While knee bends as a mobilizing and strengthening exercise are now considered undesirable, the squatting position nevertheless has some use in pregnancy and is necessary for good body mechanics in such actions as lifting in order to avoid

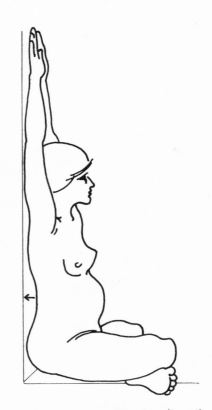

Stretch your arms and back against the wall. Keep the contact and move arms from shoulder level toward the ears.

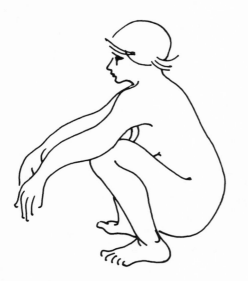

Some can squat with ease and rest elbows on knees.

stooping. The body is very stable in this position since the center of gravity is lowered. The pelvis should be tilted backward and the spine held straight. The small of the back feels very comfortable in this position, especially if you are tired, and the calf muscles benefit from a good stretch. Rest your elbows on your knees when you can balance alone. Use your knees to stand up and keep your back straight all the way from the start; don't lift up from the waist after your knees are straight. This can be awkward in later pregnancy, so start practicing as early as you can. For some people, squatting is too difficult a position to achieve or maintain and should not be forcefully pursued. Don't risk falling or hurting yourself; practice while holding on to someone or to a firm support (bed, chair, doorway), or while leaning against a wall. The feet should be flat and wide apart to avoid compression of the abdomen. The inner borders of the feet must not roll in with the arch pressed down, which happens when the knees point inside the feet instead of outward. Those with large calves may find that their legs go to sleep at first, but the circulation does improve with practice. It is helpful for beginners to wear shoes with a medium heel or to squat with the heels on a brick or piece of wood.

Others need support in the squatting position.

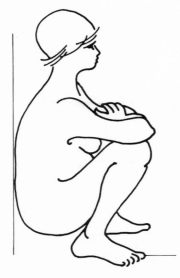

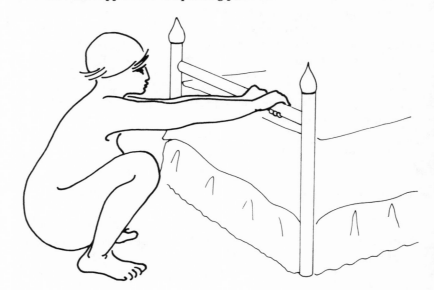

If you watch a toddler, you'll notice how easily and naturally he or she squats. As the child grows up, however, he or she learns to sit in chairs like the rest of us and in time the calf muscles tighten, the joints of the ankles and back become stiff, and a squatting position may seem very alien. In the parts of the world where people live without chairs, adults still squat. Even in some countries where there is furniture, you often find the plumbing facilities arranged so that elimination occurs in the squatting position (France, the Middle East, Asia). The human body exhibits the same physical structure everywhere; differences in its use are governed by cultural habits. A conspicuous example, where the norm varies immensely, concerns a society's approach to many aspects of pregnancy, labor, and birth. For example, squatting is the position for delivery in many countries; the pelvis is at its widest and the force of the abdominals and gravity can be well utilized. In the United States, a modified squatting position is now often used, with the back supported and propped and the legs bent and apart. Squatting (instead of leaning from the waist) while you do household work enables you to get down to floor level, to pick up things, look in the oven, lift up a child, to work in the garden, and so on with minimal strain to the back. The pelvic joints are supported yet limbered up in this position.

Stoop with ease; bend your knees.

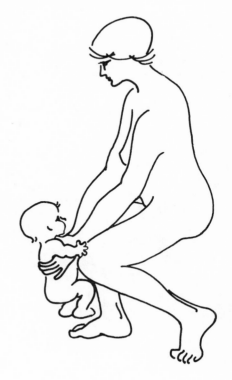

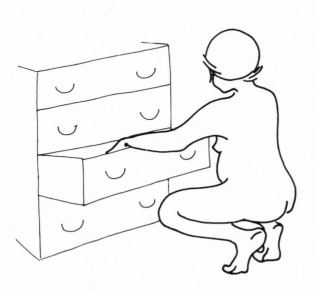

Posture in Action: Good Body Mechanics

Getting up from the Horizontal Position

As pregnancy advances, you will find it more difficult to maneuver your bulky body when arising in the morning or standing up when you have been resting or exercising at floor level. Avoid jack-knifing into a sitting position — such strain on your abdominals can encourage or increase separation of the recti muscles, particularly if your abdominals are not strong and you cannot do a curl-up anyway. Furthermore, the circulation slows down when you recline. Always take care to get up slowly so that you don't feel dizzy or faint. It's a good idea to fully stretch first a couple of times with a deep breath or two.

The most comfortable and protective method of getting up is illustrated below. Bend both knees and roll them to one side, then push off with the arms so that you rise to a sitting position. Place your legs over the edge of the bed and slowly straighten the legs to stand. This way you allow the circulation to readjust itself and you don't strain muscles by jerky effort. When rising from the floor, push yourself onto one knee, using your arm for support.

Instead of jack-knifing to a sitting position, bend your knees, roll over, and use your arms and legs.

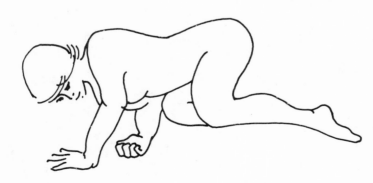
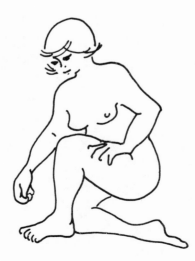

Walking

All the features of good erect posture (page 163) should be maintained as you walk. Common faults, however, include watching your feet, which results in a forward-leaning posture; rounded shoulders, with head and neck poked out in front; and a side-to-side waddle, where legs are swung sideways rather than brought straight forward from the hip. It takes some time and effort to correct any bad habits you may have developed. The easiest way is to concentrate on the key areas — head, pelvis, feet — perhaps just one at a time to begin with.

Try to tune into your posture in movement; ask those around you to watch and criticize. Keep imagining that invisible thread pulling your head up toward the ceiling as you tuck your buttocks under and place your feet, heel first, one in front of the other rather than shifting them from side to side. Beware of the tendency to sway back from the waist, to carry the pelvis forward, and to hollow the back to counter the increased weight in front. This posture will only emphasize the waddling motion already mentioned, as well as set up the vicious circle of back-strain, muscle weakness, and increased forward displacement of the pelvis and its contents. The exercises recommended will improve your muscle control so that better posture follows in all activities.

Climbing Stairs

Don't use your arms to pull yourself up steps! The handrail should be used for balance. The legs must be the force that propels your body weight upward. Place each foot firmly and completely on each step, push off from the back foot by straightening the front knee and lifting yourself up with the strong thigh and buttock muscles. Take a step at a time if necessary and don't hold your breath as you step up. Hug any packages close to your body and support them from underneath rather than at the sides. Incline your body forward as you go up but keep your body weight over the base of your feet when descending. Postpartum, you may find stairs very tiring to ascend. Take them slowly, using the propulsive power of the legs while you brace the abdominals, buttocks, and pelvic floor.

Lifting "Lift with ease . . . bend the knees"

Your back is not a crane and you should not lean forward from the waist during pregnancy to lift objects, particularly heavy ones. If you do not lower your center of gravity, you are less stable because the weaker back muscles have to pay out or lengthen. Then they must shorten from this inefficient position of stretch to raise your trunk back up again. This action is even more harmful in pregnancy with the increased vulnerability of the spinal joints and extra weight of the torso. We have all watched the way weight lifters do it: how they set the muscles and, with controlled timing, thrust upward by straightening their knees. (Your knees have much stronger muscles than your back.) Take the trouble to observe the members of your family over the next few days to see how, probably automatically, they lean over to pick up toys, other children, shopping bags, to look in low cupboards, and so on. Most people really don't lift correctly until they get a back problem.

In pregnancy your instability is increased with the forward center of gravity, softening of joints and ligaments, and — if you are wearing them — shoes with high heels. The pelvic floor also registers strain from lifting, as you will feel in pregnancy and postpartum. Get into the right lifting habits now if you have not done so before — and make sure your family reinforces them by reminding you and setting an example themselves. Heavy lifting should be passed on to someone else during the childbearing year. Don't you be the one to put out the garbage and lug suitcases at a time when you are already carrying, or recovering from, an extra load. Divide up bulky supplies and place them on lower shelves. Reaching high, for moderate or heavy objects, hollows and strains the back. If you have to lift a heavy object, protect your balance by placing your feet apart in a lunge position (see page 111). When you have to pick up from low levels or the floor, assume a squatting position — it's easier with one foot a little in front of the other. Keep your back *straight* and come *up from the knees;* don't straighten your legs and then come up from the waist! Children who want to be picked up can be encouraged to climb onto a stool or step so that you don't have to squat down so low.

When you do have to lift heavy objects, remember:

- Stand close to the load and carry it close to your body.
- Divide up loads so that you carry them equally on each side.
- Have a firm footing; one foot in front of the other in a lunge position is easier when you are lifting with the opposite arm. Feet parallel for large objects requiring both arms.

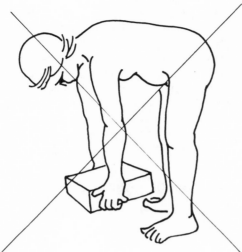

Don't crack your back.

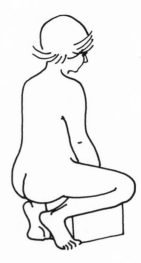

LEGS are for lifting.

- Bend your knees, *not* your back.
- Take a steady grip. Don't jerk.
- Brace the abdomen and pull up the pelvic floor, as you exhale.
- Rise up, straightening the knees. Face the direction of movement. Don't twist the trunk. Shift feet if the object turns out to be heavier than you thought.
- Move the object with a sideways lunge rather than an upward lift.

Don't make a habit of twisting your spine.

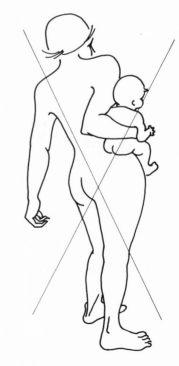

Carrying Your Baby

Supporting your baby on one hip causes your spine to twist in compensation. Similarly, carrying your baby over one shoulder increases a lumbar curve.

In recent years, many carrying aids have appeared on the market, so now we can enjoy the advantages that most women always have in other cultures. The mother's hands are liberated, and her baby feels the reassurance of her warmth and body motion. Being upright, especially after feedings, aids your baby's digestion and allows him or her to see more of the world. It must be so boring for a baby to lie flat most of the time, especially after meals (which we wouldn't like), or to see only the hood on a stroller or carriage!

Back packs or supportive slings are the most comfortable for the parent to wear. However, for the first few months, until the baby gains head control, he or she will have to be carried in a front pack. You will need to do some extra rotating exercises for the shoulder and upper back muscles to avoid fatigue. In African societies babies are carried most of the time on their mothers' back; this prevents both parties from being anxious about the whereabouts or state of the other. Babies carried this way rarely cry; nor is this spoiling them, which is a concern to some parents. Back packs also ensure good body mechanics. The wearer must bend the knees while lifting or stooping forward, otherwise the contents fall over the head!

Wheeling Strollers, Utility Carts, Supermarket Carriages

These aids are great and minimize a lot of strain and lifting if used correctly. Take care to buy a stroller or baby carriage with the handle at the proper height. If the handle is too low, you will have to lean toward it, and this should be avoided. Push the groceries along in the supermarket with the carriage held close to you — not as in the sketch below.

Equipment you wheel should be high and close.

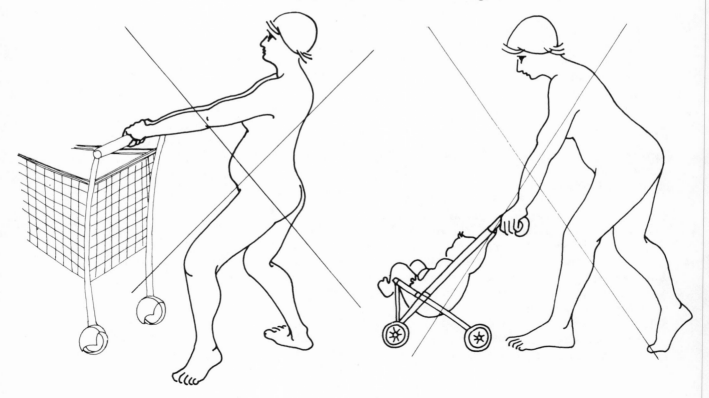

Doing Household Chores

Vacuuming, Mopping, Sweeping, Raking Leaves, Shoveling Snow

These activities involve long-levered tools, which can be tiring for the arm using them. Turn these tasks into a beneficial exercise for the abdominal and back muscles: work diagonally in a lunge position. Footwork is the key to performing these movements with ease, comfort, and grace. As a tennis player puts the left foot forward to serve with the right arm, you should use the same principle with household equipment. (Reverse if you are left-handed.) Bend the forward knee a little, as you thrust from the straightened back leg. This makes the work easier because you swing your weight back and forth into the movement instead of standing alongside the tool with one arm doing all the work and your trunk muscles held in prolonged contraction, which soon brings on fatigue.

When moving furniture, employ the same position, and bend at the knees and hips a little to line up with the object. Keep your back straight, bend your elbows, and push with both hands. The force is provided by your body weight as you thrust forward from the back foot, which assists the arms. Pushing and pivoting movements are easier than pulling and lifting ones. If you bend your knees and lower your trunk, you economize on effort, and the objects are less likely to topple over.

Exercise while you work. Use the lunge position.

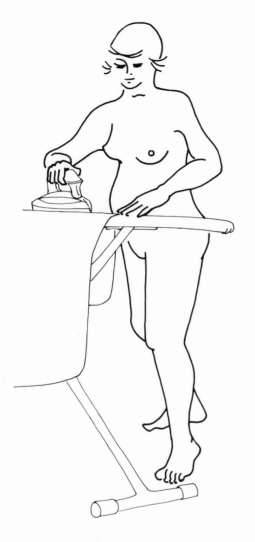

Move back and forth with your feet apart.

Working on Surfaces

If you are working at a counter, desk, ironing board, table, or similar flat surface, make sure that the height is adequate for you to work comfortably. The surface ideally should be near the level of your hip bone — so that you work with elbows bent at an angle of about 30 to 40°.

Since the sink is always lower than these surfaces, you can try washing dishes in a basin supported on another basin that is turned upside down. This will prevent your having to lean over.

Don't fold clothes on a bed. It's the fastest way to get a backache!

Use a high stool where possible, perching on the seat if you are moving back and forth a lot. Remember to place your feet so that you have both a firm base and the freedom to move backward and forward in the direction of the arms and trunk when standing at the ironing board or when cleaning furniture. Resting one foot, alternately, on a low stool or drawer helps prevent backache when standing.

Kneel or squat when you wash the floor, clean the bathtub, or wash a child.

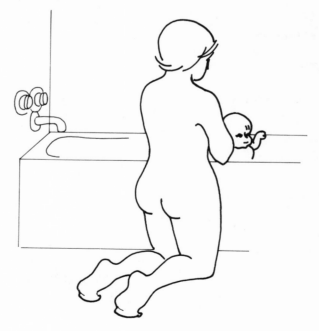

Kneel like this. Don't lean over the bathtub.

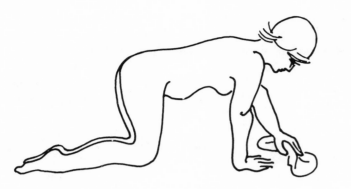

Work on all fours instead of bending up and down.

Artificial Supports

Corsets in pregnancy and binders postpartum are not recommended since they give your natural corset — the abdominal muscles — a vacation. Allowing the muscles to remain passive retards their return to normal function. Pantyhose were a great invention and have liberated us from suspender belts and other forms of foundation garments. If you feel comfortable in light elastic pants, which do *not* substitute for abdominal muscle work, it's fine to wear them. Just make sure that they do not fit too tightly, especially around the legs, as this could interfere with circulation. In rare cases a maternity girdle may be medically prescribed for support in pregnancy if obesity, twins, or extreme spinal curvature cause back pain. Likewise, after the birth an abdominal binder would be necessary only where there is severe muscle weakness, such as that which prevents the mother from raising her head and shoulders more than a couple of inches off the bed. But it must be understood that this support is only very temporary; it is a splint to assist in restoring the muscles to their normal strength.

On the other hand, a *bra* is strongly recommended — whatever your feelings are concerning women's liberation! There are *no* muscles in the breast, contrary to what you may read elsewhere (although exercises for the muscles lying beneath the breasts are often given to improve circulation and lactation).

During pregnancy, the familiar factors of increasing weight and gravity apply to the breasts in the same way as they affect the uterus and pelvic floor. Unless support is provided, the breast tissue will stretch and the bustline will sag. A well-fitting bra improves your posture and can minimize upper backache from the weight of the breasts. If your breasts are particularly large and full, it may be more comfortable for you to wear a bra to bed as well.

Make sure that the bra you select has broad straps and provides stability and support. Don't buy one that makes you feel bouncy or suspended, or with elastic straps which do not last. Check also to make sure it is not too tight for proper circulation. There is a great variety of styles in nursing bras for breast-feeding mothers, but buy these after delivery so that you get the best fit and support.

Take care when you breast-feed that your baby is not held so low that he or she drags down on the breast because this will stretch the tissues. Rather than rounding your shoulders forward, use a pillow on your lap to bring the baby a little higher or place your foot on a low stool or the rung of a chair to raise your thigh (see page 92).

While the pumping action of muscle exercise is the best way to improve the return of blood from the legs, elastic support stockings may be needed for comfort and to help varicose veins. For best results, elevate your legs while you put them on before arising in the morning since your legs have been horizontal all night and swelling and congestion is less than after you stand. Socks or knee-highs with tight elastic tops are as bad as garters in interfering with the blood circulation in the legs, and must always be avoided in pregnancy.

If the veins of the vulva become distended and painful, a perineal pad can be worn for support and comfort. All these measures, however, treat the symptoms — not the cause. The preventive approach uses exercise, changes in position, and other comfort measures so that these pregnancy-related problems are less likely to occur.

Exercises to Improve Posture

EXERCISE 1: STRETCH OUT THE KINKS

This exercise has its greatest use in later pregnancy and immediate postpartum when you want to work the back and abdominal

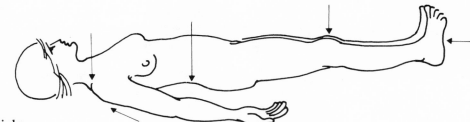

Stretch out the kinks.

muscles with minimal leverage on the joints. After delivery your body has to readjust suddenly to the loss of weight; it's easiest to start training in the horizontal position, before you take on the force of gravity.

Position: Lying on back, arms at sides, palms up, legs out straight.

Action: Bend up feet toward you to stretch calves as you press knees into the bed. Try to flatten the hollow in your back by pulling in the abdominals, and to press out the curve in the back of the neck, pulling shoulder blades together. Hold this stretched position for a few seconds and relax.

Progression: Standing or sitting against the wall. See pages 86 and 103.

EXERCISE 2: PELVIC TILTING

This essential exercise for posture control in pregnancy and postpartum was discussed in the last chapter, pages 67–74.

EXERCISE 3: BRIDGING

Bridging, or raising the hips from the floor, exercises the muscles of the buttocks which, with the abdominals, control the pelvic tilt. They need to work hard in pregnancy and postpartum as the abdominals become stretched and less able to do their share. The buttocks muscles are well developed in humans since we sit on them, and they work strongly in running, jumping, and climbing stairs, although not in ordinary walking. They extend the hips when we get up from chairs or the floor, providing an antigravity thrust. The buttocks muscles also contribute to erect posture in standing.

The circulation in the legs also benefits from such exercise, since the main muscle of the buttocks exerts a pumping effect on the veins through its attachment to the thigh. Furthermore, strengthening this muscle will provide additional support for the back of the pelvis; it attaches there and blends with one of the ligaments.

Tensing the buttocks, tucking under the seat during pelvic-tilting and posture correction, will exercise the muscles. In the following position they work strongly to lift the body weight against gravity.

Position: Lying on back, feet elevated on low stool, end of bed, or coffee table.

Action: Contract abdominal wall and buttocks and raise hips off the floor so that trunk and legs are in a straight line. Do *not* arch the back by trying to raise beyond this point. Hold

Raise the hips to form a bridge.

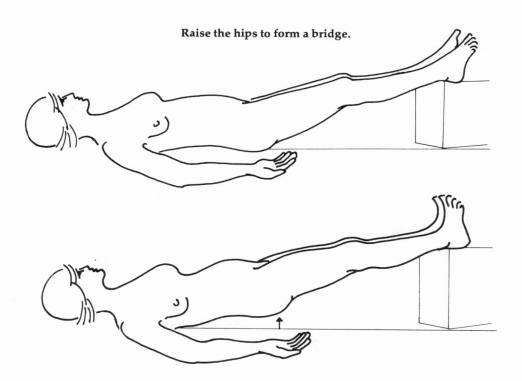

a few seconds, then slowly lower. The pelvic floor can also be contracted during this exercise. Postpartum, it is very important to close the sphincters as tightly as possible and clench the buttocks to protect the perineum from gaping.

While you are in the hospital postpartum, you will find it more practical to do this exercise in bed.

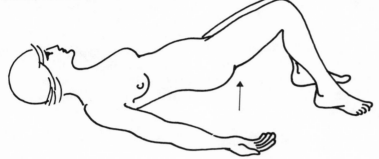

Position: Lying on back, knees bent.

Action: Raise hips so that knees and chest form a straight line. The closer the feet are to the buttocks, the more leverage you achieve; however, do *not* arch the back because you will strain the ligaments and stretch the abdominals. Contracting both abdominals and buttocks together should prevent this and keep the pelvis stable. This exercise also helps to prevent tightness in the muscles at the front of the hips. Progress by moving your feet farther away from your buttocks. Always pull the buttocks together as tightly as you can, so that you lift with these muscles rather than the hamstrings in the back of thighs.

Progression: Raise buttocks with one knee bent and the other straightened in line with the thigh — no higher. Exhale as you raise.

Progress the bridging exercise by raising the body weight with one leg.

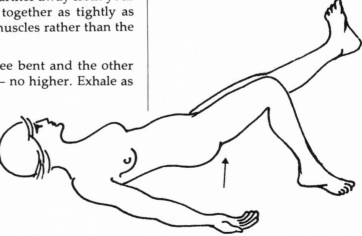

Foot Exercises

The movement of frequent foot-bending and -stretching and ankle-rotating provides a venous pump to assist the return of blood from the lower legs, and will minimize varicosities and swelling of the ankles. Cramps, which often occur from lack of exercise, may be relieved. When moving the feet, hold your legs still; this will work the thigh muscles statically and localize the movement in the feet and ankles instead of allowing the legs to roll haphazardly in and out. The small muscles in the front of the foot are strengthened by the action of raising up the arch underneath the ball of the foot while the toes are kept *straight.* Foot exercises relieve pain and adjust the muscles to increasing weight incurred during pregnancy so that deformities are prevented.

EXERCISE 4: FOOT-BENDING AND FOOT-STRETCHING

Position: Sitting or lying. In either position, legs can be relaxed over a pillow or the feet can be elevated. At other times, rest foot on the opposite knee. (This makes it easier to see your feet late in pregnancy!) It's also a good way to put on socks or pantyhose. Sitting with the legs out straight provides additional stretch of the calf muscles.

Action: Bend the ankle as far as you can, pulling your toes up toward you, thus stretching the calf muscles; then point the foot downward, making an arch. Do this several times and take a short rest before repeating. If pointing the foot results in cramps, just stretch up . . . relax . . . stretch up.

This is an easy exercise to perform throughout the day whenever you are sitting. It can also be done when you stand, but be sure to keep contact with something firm in case you lose your balance.

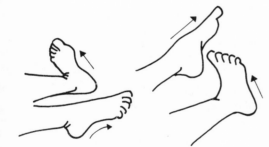

Bend and stretch your feet at the ankles.

EXERCISE 5: ANKLE-ROTATING

Position: As for Exercise 4, and any time you're off your feet.

Action: Make large slow circles with each foot, first in a clockwise, then in a counterclockwise direction. You can do both feet together, or move them in opposite directions, or rotate one at a time. Some people have difficulty coordinating the feet, so start off rotating one foot at a time if that's easier.

Note: Both foot-bending and -stretching and ankle-rotating keep things moving if you are confined to bed for any reason. These exercises are very important postpartum to prevent thrombosis — particularly if you've had general anesthesia for a caesarean section or other complications — but need not be continued once you are walking around again.

Calf-Stretching

Since cramps are so common in pregnancy and can often be brought on simply by pointing the feet down (as in the previous exercise), calf-stretching can be tried as a preventive measure.

1. Active calf-stretching in the lunge position: Stand with one foot well in front of the other. Keep back leg straight and heel on floor. Gradually bend the front knee and lean your weight

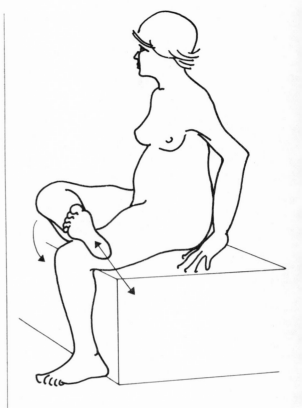

Rotate your feet — in, out, one at a time, together.

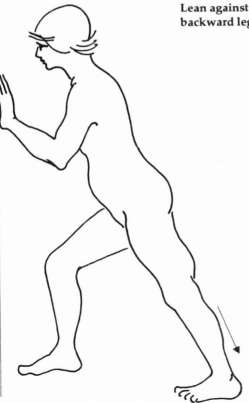

Lean against the wall and stretch the backward leg.

on to it, without raising the back heel from the floor. Take a wider stance to increase the stretch. (Squatting also exerts a stretch on part of the calf muscles.)

2. Passive calf-stretching with the help of someone else: While your leg is outstretched and relaxed, your partner should grasp the heel in his or her hand and, with a forearm under your foot, force the foot upward as far as your ankle permits. When the foot has reached this limit, your partner should press down on the knee, without losing the position of the ankle, and, if possible, periodically exert some gentle pressure at your foot to provide intermittent stretching of your calf muscles. It is important that this repeated pressure increase the stretch slightly, from stretch to stretch-plus. Take care not to release the tautness gained by the fixed positions of the ankle and knee. Stretching out cramped muscles aids the circulation, and improved circulation often means fewer cramps. A small towel or facecloth placed under the knee joint will protect it from being strained if you have loose joints. Best results are obtained when the stretching is done routinely for about 5 minutes in the evening and in the morning.

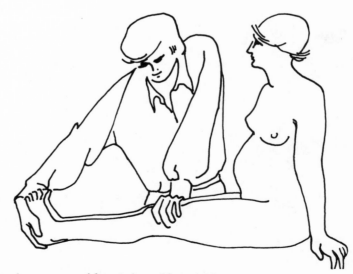

A partner can provide passive calf-stretching.

5 Relaxation

ANY EXERCISE PROGRAM, like one's daily life, should include periods of rest and relaxation. Rest is nonactivity, and, like sleep, is essential. Even your heart, which rhythmically beats for the whole of your life, rests more than it works. Fatigue interferes not only with the ability of muscles to contract, but also to relax. For this reason, we may experience cramps when certain muscles are working overtime and waste products accumulate in them. Muscles can be overloaded in more subtle yet far-reaching ways, such as the persistence of generalized body tension without release, which builds up stress in all the body systems. Effective relaxation, which reverses these detrimental effects, is essential for good health.

Relaxation is more than just rest and stillness. For some people the term conveys the idea of doing nothing, napping, or sitting back and being entertained. But, in fact, genuine relaxation requires that we gain insight into our muscular system, with which we make all purposeful actions in life and express our emotions. It involves learning to recognize, and release, excess tension, which may be present although the muscles are performing no activity. Research has shown that people can become aware of their levels of muscular tension and learn to lower them. Even monkeys have been successfully trained to control their muscle tension to a very specific degree.

States of tension within the body can become habitual without our being aware of it, since our conscious levels adapt readily. Even at rest, opposing muscles are always in balance; if tension is increased in one group, equivalent tension will be invoked in another. In this way, levels of residual tension at rest can vary tremendously between individuals. The misuse of energy — tension — can be localized in a certain area, such as the neck, or the effects can become more pervasive and cumulative, causing changes in posture, habits, and personality. Unnecessary "bracing" of voluntary muscles causes a simultaneous "alerting" of the nervous system and vice versa. This vicious circle of stress is one of the dangerous threats of

Western life. Because the pernicious adjustments to stress demand such a price in strokes and heart attacks (accounting for more than half the deaths each year in the United States), much interest has been generated in recent years concerning ways to relieve stress and lower blood pressure.

While yoga and other techniques for meditation and relaxation have been practiced in various places for centuries, some significant developments have occurred in the last decade that have been popularly received in this country. These techniques — namely, biofeedback theory, transcendental meditation or its modification, the "relaxation response" — are not complicated, and they provide rapid results that have been scientifically verified.

Biofeedback theory involves the lowering of muscle tension as the result of conscious voluntary control. Since the highly sensitive monitoring equipment feeds back the minutest degrees of tension, it is possible for attention to be focused on even the smallest unit of a muscle. While this process requires considerable motivation, the individual is accurately and continuously informed of his or her progress, and it takes a very short time — sometimes less than an hour — for amazing control to be exerted over muscle tension. Unlike transcendental meditation, the activity is direct, specific, and purposeful, achieving on-going measurable results.

Transcendental meditation or the relaxation response is much simpler in that no equipment is required and the technique can be performed in any place of quiet and comfort. However, it may take several weeks for this process to cause a significant decrease in stress. Repetition is involved in improving the response, and the effects occur indirectly since the individual remains passive. Release of stress occurs in a state of "restful alertness" (which is quite different from sleep), and benefits several physiological functions in addition to muscle tension.

Just as there are various methods for achieving relaxation, techniques can be modified to suit the needs of an individual with regard to time and place. Passive relaxation is a way of taking a break from the outside world, whereas active relaxation enables us to function with calm efficiency in coping with a particular stress situation. The interesting feature common to these current techniques is that people gain the skill and benefits of relaxation independently, through their own self-direction. No pill, prescription, or other external agent is required. Relaxation is free, always available, and is far more effective than any drug or stimulant in regenerating one's total being. Instead of falling victim to our psychosomatic processes we learn awareness and autonomy so we can modify them.

Passive relaxation occurs when the individual temporarily withdraws into the bubble of his or her private world. Release pervades the whole body because the mind is neither reflecting nor analyzing. Instead of trying to force the mind to remain blank, a mental state of low arousal is achieved passively. This process is enhanced by repeating a simple word or a meaningless sound, such as a mantra, listening to music, fantasizing a peaceful rural scene, or focusing on one's breathing rhythm. Thoughts are allowed to pass in and out of the mind, but one's mental attitude remains quite passive to any idea or emotion. Most people share the opinion that an ideal amount of time to practice passive relaxation is about 20 minutes. Initially, it may be difficult for a goal-oriented person accustomed to "purposeful" activity to feel comfortable being alone with her or his self, doing "nothing." It is essential not to anticipate or make plans for the end of the session while attempting to relax! The process is similar to attaining orgasm. In both states it is important to release the mind and the body; as long as you continue to spectate and evaluate how you are getting along, participation is blocked. Of course, in the beginning one is always a little tense with wanting to perform well. As self-consciousness diminishes, self-confidence increases so that it becomes easy to let go.

Relaxation can also be done during brief opportunities, such as in a traffic jam or during a coffee break. A quick release of body tensions with your head dropped forward is an instant refresher. (At first the muscles and ligaments at the back of your neck may protest if they are tight from maintaining the head constantly in an erect position. They will lengthen with practice and discomfort in this area, commonly felt by commuters and desk workers, will be relieved.)

Active relaxation differs from the passive form by involving interaction with the environment without undue tension or muscle expenditure. All of us have experienced occasions when our nervous system seems more excitable than usual, and a barking dog or honking horn causes us to jump abruptly. Regular practice of passive relaxation benefits many organs and systems within the body so that the nervous system operates at lower levels of arousal, but we also need to cultivate the ability to be mentally attentive while simultaneously relaxing the parts of the body that are extraneous to the task at hand, such as when driving in traffic or performing a skill. Active relaxation involves identification of tense areas in the body. Clues are provided by posture, work habits, and parts of the body that feel tired and stiff. Movements, such as stretching or shaking, help you to consciously recognize the contrasting states of tension and relaxation. Reversing habitual patterns of muscle contraction results in lengthening, that is, relaxation, of the tight muscle groups. Active relaxation can include the whole body or simply focus on key areas, like the neck or jaw, at brief intervals during the day. Preparation for labor and delivery is assisted by the use of physical techniques to achieve relaxation because this is a time of stress when the physical involuntary nature of the events is most significant. Athletes must also learn how to effectively relax — particularly since they are primarily concerned with body-building through progressive muscular contraction.

The tension that all relaxation techniques aim to alleviate concerns the state of readiness of the muscles for a situation of sudden action or emotion — when such a state does not exist. Tension serves a useful purpose in such cases: it prepares the body for action — for "fight or flight." But if it is allowed to persist when the need is no longer there, it may become habitual and interfere with rest and sleep. We have all seen these tense types: face "set," shoulders hunched, arms folded, knees crossed. There may be irregular breathing, a tapping foot, or other nervous gestures. People exhibiting these signs can even alter the tension levels of those around them! Gaining skills in relaxation pays off with greater poise and emotional serenity as well as such physiological benefits as reduced blood pressure (since better circulation is allowed when the muscles are free from undue tension). With bodily tensions reduced, there are fewer cramped muscles, headaches, backaches, and insomnia. Learning this art — learning to unwind — is of value for the rest of our lives, whatever our age, sex, or occupation.

Relaxation During Pregnancy

During pregnancy, the body is in a different and changing physiological condition, which also affects one's psychological state. Discomfort, bizarre dreams, ambivalence concerning the pregnancy, fear about the development and safety of the baby, distress at the inevitability of the life process, concern for changes in the marital relationship, or feelings of inadequacy regarding one's ability to be a parent — these are all normal experiences causing anxiety in women during pregnancy. Superstitions and "fear of failure" in labor can increase any apprehension that may be felt. Some women feel guilty and depressed, thinking (mistakenly) that no one else would share these thoughts and feelings, and so they repress them instead of venting them. The physician rarely has the time to discuss such matters, and the baby's father is probably experiencing a similar set of worries. In fact, since fatherhood has no outward visible signs, a father, in our culture, tends to be overlooked until the arrival of the child — and may be undergoing a greater psychological crisis. Regular relaxation helps to reduce the emotional stress that accumulates with focusing too much on "D-Day."

It is hard to relax the body — whatever method you use — when the mind is not at ease. Work toward achieving both goals. Read and learn what you can, attend classes that discuss parenthood, childbearing, and so on; knowledge is the best way to gain self-assurance and faith in one's body during this natural process. Practicing the physical steps toward relaxation can also help to release the mind. The body systems interact so perfectly that, just as the mind can control the state of the muscles, so tension in the muscles can alter other states of the body through a subconscious part of our nervous system. Although the mind is the dominant center of control, by attaining relaxation in the voluntary muscle system we can influence relaxation in the involuntary muscles and other systems of the body.

It is necessary to learn relaxation in pregnancy to meet not only the stresses of that state but also to prepare for a time of immense stress — labor and delivery. While the muscles in the uterus, like those in your heart, will perform their job without your conscious control, you can assist by ensuring that the muscles under your control do not become tense and thus interfere with the process. Instead, they must be relaxed. This will also mean that your energy is conserved for later, when you may need it for pushing. By learning to relax now, you will have a useful tool for release when life gets more complicated — and it will — by your need to meet the demands of an extra person, whether it is your first or fifth baby.

Those readers who have been accustomed to regular yoga, meditation, or other forms of relaxation will, of course, continue to experience benefits during the maternity cycle. Yoga and meditative techniques require much practice and trust in your body for you to be able to let your mental and physical resistance go as you confront the contractions of labor. At present, few of us have access to the sophisticated apparatus that provides technical biofeedback, although equipment that measures muscle activity or skin temperature as an index of relaxation is becoming cheaper and more available. Pulse readings can also be taken for biofeedback. Sometimes it's preferable to have this done by someone else since this activity itself is often sufficient to raise the pulse rate!

Physical stretching exercises, to the point of pain, are helpful in learning to let go, although the success of relaxation ("trying not to try") depends on mental attitude. Body-awareness techniques can be progressed to provide training for coordination of muscle release with labor contractions, without sensations of stretching and pain. Human feedback may be provided by a partner who also becomes more personally involved in the childbearing preparation. This person assists by evaluating the state of tension in various muscles when checking limpness of your limbs and your response to touching, stroking, massage, and such. Practice this on each other so that you become trusting and adept in the gentle handling of each other's body.

Preparation for Relaxation

Relaxation is best practiced after an exercise session, when the muscles are slightly fatigued. It is important to slow down gradually — from activity to rest to relaxation. Without this gradual slowing down, waste products will accumulate in the body and will make the muscles ache or feel stiff later.

Lie or sit in a completely supported position of total comfort (see Chapter 4, pages 88–100, for various options). All parts of the body must be supported; if they are not, gravity will stimulate any dangling extremity to do muscle work. This includes your hands and feet in particular. Gravity has the least stimulating effect on the body when you are lying down, on the back, front, side, or three-quarters over. In sitting or half-lying positions there will be less resistance under the diaphragm from the abdominal contents, so these positions may be preferable in later pregnancy. Since we spend so much of our time sitting, it is essential — and for some busy mothers more practical — to rehearse their techniques in this position. Don't overlook obvious points, such as being adequately warm, having the clothing loose and shoes off, and making sure that the general atmosphere is conducive to relaxation.

The supporting surface should be firm. If it sags, then support will be lost and positions of strain can be created (particularly the back if the mattress hollows in the middle, for example). Use as many cushions and pillows as you need to accommodate completely body curves and to relieve all pressure points. Large bean-bag chairs can be very satisfactory. Resilient foam or rubber pillows may interfere with relaxation; they often cause or aggravate neck tension. A feather pillow or kapok cushion does not require continual adjustment of the joints, as does a springy surface. Instead, you just let the head sink right down into it.

Check that all joints are slightly bent; this relieves the mechanical tension that activates the body's stretch reflex (preparing the muscles for action). You are aiming for the opposite state: repose and release.

Individuals vary greatly in their ability to relax. Some people are able to release with such ease that they have no need of further instruction. Others always have a kind of battle with the process, which is quite self-defeating. The large majority in the middle can really improve their relaxation skills by creating the right conditions and undertaking regular practice and progression. There is certainly no reason why a person could not or should not learn the art of relaxation. Techniques which enable one's performance to be checked may be more encouraging than attempting more subtle ways of gaining body awareness at first. Similarly it is easier to learn to relax under the most favorable conditions before trying it in waiting rooms or on public transport.

Techniques for Relaxation

Muscle work always has at least two parts to it. A muscle contracts and shortens or it relaxes and lengthens. In this way muscles also work together — but in an exactly opposite relationship, which is reciprocal. For example, when we bend an elbow the biceps muscle contracts and the triceps muscle behind lengthens to allow the movement. Sometimes this interaction may be disturbed, as when your foot goes into cramp. The muscle remains in a state of contraction, which becomes painful because it is prolonged and very fatiguing. Furthermore, you are unable to work the opposite group of muscles, which bend your foot upward, without applying some extra force to stretch out passively the cramped muscle. Normally, however, you can freely move your foot up, shortening those muscles while the neighbors relax, or point your foot down, relaxing the first group and contracting the second.

Relaxation is the physiological state that follows muscle contraction. This principle is utilized in relaxation training. Even the simple act of breathing in and out is a natural way to experience mild tension and relaxation. Muscles contract as air is taken in, and their release allows the air to be exhaled. If you become skilled at observing your breathing, you will notice another state, of nonactivity, during the pause within the breathing cycle. It is an interesting fact that orgasm, like relaxation, cannot be forced. The mind has to allow the body to follow its own wisdom. Sexual analogies are more appropriate for the experience of labor than are the more common examples of bowel movements. Furthermore, elimination to many people means straining, which is the antithesis of relaxation.

A common approach is to use muscle contraction to make tension more obvious — for example, making a fist or shrugging your shoulders. In theory, this is supposed to provide a sense of relaxation through fatigue. However, the problem is that you are actually making tense muscles more tense. It has never been shown that this lowers the tension level that you started from. Sometimes it is helpful for your partner to see and feel a tense muscle. But it makes more sense to contract the opposite muscle group so that the tight muscles are obliged to relax according to the laws of the body. We have seen that voluntary muscles work in groups. Yoga programs have recognized this for centuries. In yoga, a movement in one direction is followed by a balance of movement in the opposite direction.

Laura Mitchell, in her excellent book, *Simple Relaxation*, has selected a few photographs that show the characteristic body language of tension. Anxiety and anger, from whatever cause, result in a typical pattern of muscle contraction and shortening. The difficulty with relaxation, as she astutely points out, is that information about muscle tension is not conveyed to the conscious brain. A simple experiment verifies this experience. Even with our eyes closed, we know if our elbow is bent, but we cannot know the state of the muscles above and below the joint. The mind knows only movements, not individual muscles. Mitchell's approach is based on the physiological principle of reciprocal relaxation. Contraction of one group necessarily results in relaxation of the opposing muscle group. Therefore, if you pull your shoulders toward your feet, the tight muscles that hunch your shoulders up to your ears are obliged to relax and lengthen. She has refined a series of specific orders to reverse classic muscle tension patterns. This indirect and effective method of relaxation can be learned by anyone. The program is clear and concise. Relaxation sessions may involve all the significant movements, or any one movement, at any time. For example, if you tend to clench your fist, or use your fingers a lot, stretching the fingers ''long'' will achieve relaxation of the tense flexor muscles.

Progressive relaxation techniques form the basis of most childbirth education classes. In England, relaxation and exercises for pregnant women were instituted as early as the 1920s. Dr. Edmund Jacobson was one of the first medical men in the USA to recognize the clinical value of relaxation. His book, *Progressive Relaxation*, published in 1929, outlined the techniques that form the basis of many childbirth education classes. In a position of comfort, all the joints in the body are worked loose in a logical progression. You experience activity, such as raising your hand, and then focus on recognizing rest or nonactivity when you cease the movement. The detailed program, which is quite time-consuming, can be found in Jacobson's book, *How to Relax and Have Your Baby*. Modifications of this approach that involve a partner are common in prenatal classes. This enables checking and stroking skills to be developed in preparation for support in labor.

In yoga, relaxation is achieved through both physical and mental techniques. The asanas, or positions, involve the body in a series of stretches. Most of these extend the parts of the body where sedentary people are tight. The challenge and rewards of yoga lie in the confrontation of these physical and mental limitations. One soon learns that forcing only increases the resistance. The joints increase their range of movement only when the mind lets go. If a difficult posture is painful, one breathes *into* the pain. (This contrasts with the Lamaze approach of dissociating and blocking out discomfort.) The mental discipline in yoga also involves meditation, the key to which is listening to the breath. However, concentrating on asanas or other activities that quiet the conscious mind also produces a meditative state that leads to calm and well-being.

Checking and Feedback

The partner starts with observing outward signs. The expectant mother's face should be expressionless and the breathing quiet and without effort. All joints must be slightly flexed and the hips should be relaxed to allow the legs to roll out so that the feet point sideways.

Next, try gently checking the extremities. Neuromuscular principles determine that release spreads out from the center, when checking work in the reverse, from the periphery, to see if relaxation has been achieved. Begin by gently raising the hand a little. If it is loose and feels heavy, this means it is relaxed. If it is stiff and light, it is *not* relaxed. Then try the joint above. Ease the elbow up and down; if you feel resistance take the whole arm next. Support it above and below the elbow and "work it loose" with a gentle slow circling motion from the shoulder joint. Let it drop back softly to check that the muscles have released and the limb is weighty. Raising the legs in such a way is too disturbing (although one leg can be raised voluntarily, as in Step 1). Rolling the thighs in and out will loosen the hip and knee. Handling the feet can be ticklish (unless done firmly); downward bending of the toes can cause cramp. Rotating the ankles or stroking the calf may also help. (Remember to watch for curling toes during labor — a classic indication of tension.)

Next, your partner can refine the process by placing his or her hands firmly on a part of your body to initiate greater relaxation of the underlying muscles. (Both hands must be placed, otherwise the subject wonders where and when the other hand will arrive and this impairs relaxation!) You attempt to release a little more when you feel the contact and warmth. Developing these nonverbal techniques reduces the need for spoken commands and is an advance in more subtle forms of control and release. Some people are also aided by the repetition of suggestive words, such as "limp," "droopy," "loose," "calm," "give," "ease," "slow," "heavy," "slack," "warm," "floating," and so on. Or these words can be used affirmatively to acknowledge and reinforce the student's success at self-direction.

Massage is a useful aid here. It will increase sensory awareness, improve circulation, relieve stiffness and discomfort — and feels wonderful. Work downwards to avoid friction against the hairs. Soothing massage of the neck and shoulders; light circling with the fingers on the muscles of the face and jaw; firm counterpressure on the small of the back for backache; light stroking of the taut abdominal area — or anywhere where it feels good to be touched. A thorough massage of the feet feels marvelous and is claimed by zone therapists to reflexly benefit the whole body. Continuity with both hands, plus firm pressure make massage relaxing rather than stimulating since muscles initially respond to touch with a slight reflex contraction.

The rhythm of slow deep breathing assists relaxation. Each time you exhale, breathe out a little more residual tension. Think "relax" as you sigh gently on outward breath, since natural relaxation occurs on exhalation. It is very important to *observe* your breathing without controlling it. This engages your conscious mind and frees your body from tension in a way that you cannot achieve directly. The more you relax, the quieter your breathing. With practice you become increasingly aware of the pause between the exhaled and incoming breaths.

The eyes may close naturally during relaxation sessions, or you may prefer to keep them loosely open. Some people like to tune in with eyes shut, others prefer to turn off by gazing vaguely at a point. Harmonizing the mind with body states is a personal experience.

Relaxation for Labor

Even the most well-prepared expectant mother feels some apprehension when the inevitable process of labor, with its unknown events which she cannot control, commences. Time passes most pleasantly with normal activities at home in the early stages. It is helpful for the progress of labor to remain upright, walking and sitting as much as is comfortable, because the drive force of the uterus is most efficient in these positions. If you are planning a hospital birth, use of the fetal monitor and/or intravenous may curtail your freedom. However, home-like birth rooms are becoming more common, as well as independent birth centers staffed by midwives committed to natural childbirth.

The labor bed is not the place to negotiate certain requests or modifications of hospital procedures. These are best discussed with the medical staff beforehand and should be documented in your chart. Probably half of the content of the child-birth preparation course is information to acquaint a couple with hospital procedures and intervention and to provide them with coping mechanisms for this environment. It is assumed that, since every labor and delivery is different for each woman, what institutional flexibility exists should be responsive to that individual's personal needs. The assembly-line approach, called "hospital policy," could be much more adaptable without re-ducing the quality of health care. In fact, the quality would be improved if women had more input and control over their birthing experience. Medical decisions, of course, must be made by qualified professionals, but the experiential value of childbirth is often overlooked. What we want is a healthy baby and mother *and* a good experience. Visiting the labor and delivery area before you need to go there, being aware of the hospital rules and routine and the various actions that can be expected from the staff will reduce some of the anxiety that can mar relaxation. Women in this country who deliver at home or in a childbearing center find relaxation much easier because they are not in the "patient role," having to contend with hos-pital policies. (They may, however, have other worries, such as whether there will be an emergency.) Childbirth is never with-out some risk, and no culture approaches this life crisis without some foreboding or ritual.

Discomfort and Pain

A supportive birth environment is important for a woman's morale and is most significant in helping her to relax. The phys-ical aspects of relaxation are intimately connected with mental states. Fear and anxiety, we all know, cause tension. Women are more suggestible in pregnancy than at other times and may readily become apprehensive. In labor they are particularly vul-nerable, not only because of the overwhelming force occurring within them, unlike anything experienced before, but also be-cause they are very dependent at this time on those around them. Self-confidence and a partner who provides positive sup-port and comfort measures are most significant at this time.

Fear and anxiety in labor cause tension, which interferes with the body's natural functions and can lead to physical dis-comfort or pain. Tension, whether you are conscious of it or not, pervades the whole body. Emotions can inhibit the activity of the uterus; contractions often stop for a short while when the mother arrives at the hospital. During labor the cervix should be quite passive, allowing the muscles of the uterus to open it up, contraction by contraction. However, if your "flight or fight" mechanisms are activated, the tension will spread to the circular muscles of the cervix and cause them to constrict. This conflicts with the work of the uterus, and antagonistic muscle work is as uncomfortable as it is unnecessary. The cervix during the first stage of labor should be like the pelvic floor during the second stage — without tension or resistance, and stretching in submission to the forces from above. It is hard to achieve this when you may be feeling tired and uncomfortable, and it will become more difficult as the contractions continue to get stronger and closer together and your fatigue increases. Understanding what is happening, and why, is essential if you are to feel motivated to trust in your body and to flow with its natural rhythms. (Information as to progress of dilatation is reassuring since you have no direct knowledge of this; it can be assessed only through a pelvic examination.)

The uterus is simply a bag of muscle that involuntarily contracts to expel its contents. There may be referred backache from the stretching of the cervix (in first stage) or the position of the baby, or discomfort may be felt from pressure on the pelvic organs (during second stage). If the reasons are understood, alarm is avoided and much of this discomfort will be considered tolerable, particularly because there are always intervals between the contractions. Often the distress may be caused not so much by the physical presence of actual pain but by a combination of fear, fatigue, and, in transition, for example, nausea and tremors when pressure against nerves can cause the legs to shake uncontrollably. On rare occasions there is real pathology and in these cases pain serves as an important warning sign.

The degrees to which some of the anticipated discomforts of labor are felt vary greatly from individual to individual and from culture to culture. Fear, we have seen, brings more pain than the pain it fears. Other significant factors, which determine the amount of pain that is felt and, most important, how it is interpreted, include culture, ethnic group, religion, past experiences, time, place, mental preoccupation, and suggestibility. Likewise, the effectiveness of drugs depends on the circumstances under which they are administered, as research with placebos has shown. If you scrape your shin in the dentist's office, it feels worse than if it happened in a hockey game, where you may not have even noticed it. If you dwell on a contraction that you "know is going to feel awful," it probably will. You may feel it less by diverting your attention elsewhere (breathing, watching your partner, massage). By being alert and staying in present time you have a psychological advantage to help cope with pain if you experience it. If you decide that the contraction is probably just muscle work and that you will tune in to figure out what the sensation involves, you may not find it painful. Considerable vocal expression of your emotions may be appropriate for your personality and culture. Individuals vary and each woman must develop her own approach to birth. Women who have been to prepared childbirth classes often feel pressure to conform and to be "in control." They are reluctant to let go and do what feels right, particularly if it is noisy or uninhibited behavior. Unfortunately, any self-restraint works in opposition to relaxation.

Many researchers have shown that labor is less painful and more efficient with help from gravity, that is, when the mother is in an upright position, walking around. Studies have also demonstrated that there is a decreased need for drugs, anesthetics, and uterine stimulants. Furthermore, less heart rate abnormalities or molding of the fetal head occur when the mother is standing and walking. Often women instinctively rock and roll the pelvis during contractions and they should be free to actively move around in whatever way feels right.

Hypnosis, acupuncture, medication, anesthesia, pressure-reducing "birth suits," and Lamaze techniques for dissociation all share in common the goal of diminishing the sensations of labor contractions. The history of civilization is also the history of the development of techniques to cope with the problem of pain. Yet what is strange is that physiological processes generally are not painful. Having a baby is not like having a tooth drilled; that is pathological. Occasionally, we may have a problem with our digestion or bowels (and typically we become much more aware of these functions in times of stress), but nature did not design the reproductive process with biblical torment in mind! If it were such a horrible experience, the world would never have become as overpopulated as it is.

Latest theories in the understanding of pain are very encouraging for those wanting to improve their mental and physical performance under stress. This involves a commitment to experience positively — in the sense of being alert and informed, not necessarily without discomfort. The Gate Control Theory of Melzack and Wall is most relevant to the features of prepared childbirth training since it supposes that the mind plays a significant role in "receiving" and interpreting bodily sensations. Messages of internal or external origin converge on a key point in the pathway, where resistance to their passage can be lowered or increased, rather like opening or closing a gate. We can actively raise the resistance to unwanted stimuli by "closing the gate" at both central and peripheral levels. Our will controls the "gate" in the brain and is influenced by selective attention, such as our concentrating on something else during a contraction. The gate in the spinal cord can be closed by messages arriving from the surface of the body, like those that come through massage or use of hot or cold packs. In this way we use simple physiological methods to close the gate or inhibit the amount of discomfort or pain that is felt.

Since pain is such a complex and devious phenomenon, its total eradication remains a problem even today. No anesthetic, for example, is totally effective and at the same time entirely safe for use in childbirth. There is a trade-off involved, and where the administration of medication or anesthesia is optional rather than routine the consumer needs to decide responsibly which tools she will use for relief of discomfort, if any are required. Planning a natural childbirth is not taking a one-way ticket. Pain-relieving drugs are always available but should be used as little as possible because of their well-known depressant effects on the baby. They also slow down the process of labor and may make it harder for the mother to stay in tune with her body. Dependence on these can be reduced by making pain *bearable*. Seeking to abolish all feeling denies the sensuality and sexuality of birth. While no one wants you to suffer, a nonexperience may be greatly regretted. Many women who were knocked out for the whole event make a determined effort to change physicians and to seek out childbirth preparation classes next time. (There will always be some, perhaps, who do want to be put right out and to receive a little package from the nursery the next day.) Studies have shown that the reality of having seen and felt it all has significant benefits for the successful bonding of the family members and the mother's postpartum adjustment.

Relaxation Techniques for Labor

Labor and delivery may be the time of hardest work and greatest stress that a woman ever experiences. However, it is not an athletic event and the value of relaxation as a component of this experience cannot be overemphasized. The greater your ability to relax, the more enjoyable you will find the event since your arousal state will be lowered and you will experience discomfort less. If you do have difficulty relaxing or if your labor is stormy, you will probably find that breathing patterns help little. Paced respiration is a useful tool for some, but unlike relaxation it consumes energy rather than conserving it.

During pregnancy you learned to relax passively, like a rag doll. You recognized the state of blissful restfulness of a released mind and body, usually in a position of recumbency and complete comfort. In labor many of these things change and you have to be more alert, but by non-striving, to maintain as complete a state of relaxation as you can. Like many women, you may have felt some internal sensations when practicing relaxation in pregnancy: either intermittent tightening of the uterus (Braxton-Hicks contractions) or movement of the baby, since when you lie still he or she usually starts to move around. (This is because the rocking motion, which soothes the baby when you move around, has ceased.) A change of position will usually cause the intermittent contractions to pass, although they provide a useful opportunity for practice.

However, when labor is established the contractions continue to progress, regardless of any modifications you may desire. Usually no one position is comfortable for long and you will feel the need to make changes. Often you must turn on your back, usually a very uncomfortable position at this time, for routine checks and examinations. Relaxing under these conditions is much more demanding than it was in pregnancy.

The stretching exercises described on pages 102–103 are helpful in learning how to give in when it hurts. Your partner should also share these experiences with you. This way you can both appreciate what relaxation involves and together can benefit from improving your abilities to relax under stress. Although the assistance and support of a partner is valuable, this body-mind work can only come from within. No one else can do it for you; they can only observe the blockages, the areas of resistance and tension.

Yoga provides excellent training for the pain of childbirth. Almost every posture provides an opportunity for you to confront your limitations. (Certain positions are not advisable during the childbearing year; see pages 16–18.) Just sitting with your legs stretched out in front may bring on an uncomfortable feeling of tightness in the hamstring muscles at the back of the knees. This can be increased if you lean forward from the waist with a straight back. Keep exhaling and moving into the pain.

You may find as you reflect on it (What color is it? Is it hot or cold, sharp or dull?) that this acceptance of the pain actually eases it. Forcing yourself to ignore it will, on the other hand, increase the resistance to movement and the sensation of discomfort.

Comfort: Use different positions and lots of pillows. Don't forget to relieve your bladder from time to time. Walking around usually makes labor shorter and less painful.

Relaxation: If your mind can stay quiet and centered, your body will have more energy. Just take each contraction as it comes.

Moral support: There's nothing like your friend or lover boosting you along with enthusiasm and encouragement.

Massage: Some women don't want to be touched at all, but others may do their own massage to occupy their hands and mind. Stroking, counterpressure, passive pelvic-rocking, and the like are very useful. Like scratching an itch, rubbing where it hurts makes the sore place feel better. It also serves to involve your partner physically and emotionally.

Heat and cold: Hot or cold packs relieve local symptoms and stimulate the nerves that send messages to help close the gate in the spinal cord. It is refreshing to wipe your face with either a hot or cold facecloth.

Breathing: Haphazard breathing benefits neither mother nor baby: take care not to hyperventilate. Your breath should flow with the contraction. Any control of the breath works against the body's equilibrium, limits feeling, and impairs relaxation. Vocal sounds — singing, moaning, chanting — should be encouraged if they help keep the breathing physiological.

Relaxation During Labor — Second Stage

Your role, when dilation is complete, is actively to assist the uterus in pushing the baby down the birth canal while remaining relaxed in the legs, face, and jaw. However, there will be longer intervals for you to rest between these contractions than you perhaps experienced in transition. For these few minutes you can relax quite passively, as you did between contractions in the first stage, although you may shiver from heat loss or experience quivering of muscles from the effort of pushing and from pressure on the nerves. Always relax until your body directs you to push. If the breath is released, rather than held, the pelvic floor will not be tensed. During the actual birth you will breathe the baby out with light pants or groans so that the pelvic floor will stretch easily. Giving birth is letting go.

Relaxation Postpartum

You will probably feel quite euphoric after the delivery, when you have held your baby and exchanged congratulations. Rest or sleep is often difficult at such a time of exhilaration — but this high is temporary. After all, your body has worked incredibly hard and has undergone some very sudden changes; you will certainly feel tired later. As in the second stage, after birth the legs often tremble because of the body's heat loss (and delivery rooms are cold) as well as muscle fatigue.

Fatigue is one of the most common complaints in this period although you will suffer less from exhaustion if you relaxed effectively during labor. In the first week, your mind, body, and daily life experience very profound adjustments. The uterus, which took nine months to grow to term, starts its six-week shrinking process, the breasts will start producing milk around the third day, and many of these hormonal changes may make you feel overwhelmed and depressed. Part of this is also the result of the anticlimax that follows any enormously important event. After you get home you may experience another low as the glamour of motherhood seems to evaporate with the demands of being both a wife and a mother, and the feeling that all your energy and time is tied to the baby.

Continuing relaxation at this time is even more important than before. Now that you will have fewer uninterrupted moments to yourself, you must gain the greatest value from them. Sitting, in general, may provide opportunities for relaxation during this busy time, although lying on your front should also be continued for a few weeks. Your baby's feeding sessions, when established, provide an opportunity for you to rest in a comfortable position, when your feet are up and you can release tension. Discomfort may be experienced during the shrinking contractions of the uterus, mostly by women who have had more than one child, since the uterus has to work harder to regain its original size. These are just muscular contractions, although they — like labor contractions — unfortunately have become synonymous with the word *pain* and are also known as "afterpains." Breast-feeding stimulates the uterus and so increases their intensity.

You must have rest and relaxation to complement the exercise program in order to renew your strength and vigor. Don't let domestic activities and chores stifle these sessions at the time when they are most needed. If your partner can take over domestic duties or a few days off work to ease the adjustments, your first week or so at home will be much smoother, especially if there are other children. Let visitors do odd jobs for you and make sure that you are not concerned with appearances or other unimportant matters at this time.

The childbearing cycle includes three months postpartum before the mind and body have reached a state of adjustment. How well you look and feel at the end of it will be the reward for your efforts.

Breathing

THIS FUNDAMENTAL ACTIVITY is emphasized by just about every school of thought concerned with improving body performance: yoga, athletics, meditation, relaxation training, and childbirth preparation classes. Some of you may be attending childbirth preparation classes in which breathing techniques are included. Nevertheless, it falls within the scope of this manual to examine the role of this vital body function in pregnancy, labor, and postpartum.

Breathing During Pregnancy

It is essential to develop a pattern of efficient breathing in pregnancy, as your body is having to cope with an increased load. The blood volume becomes enlarged to supply the growing baby with oxygen and nutrients and to excrete its carbon dioxide. While these natural adjustments of the body provide for adequate oxygen for you both and for the working muscles, the decreased movement of the respiratory muscles with the increasing pressure growing within the abdomen can cause congestion and discomfort. Learning good breathing habits has many benefits: circulation will be improved, breathlessness avoided, and the heart and lungs will be better prepared to function well in labor. Expectant mothers who suffer from chronic bronchitis, asthma, or even a cold in the last trimester, feel great discomfort. They must make a special effort to improve lung function with breathing exercises.

Deep breathing can be combined with activities and exercises; certainly you should not hold your breath! Exercises involving the shoulders and elevation of the rib cage are most suitable for conscious breathing, and will help relieve indigestion or heartburn and improve the postural sense (see pages 102–103). The form of deep breathing that is most often taught — for pregnancy and labor, before and after operations, and for lung and chest dysfunction — is diaphragmatic breathing. This

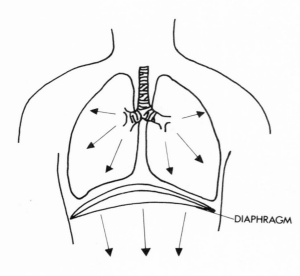

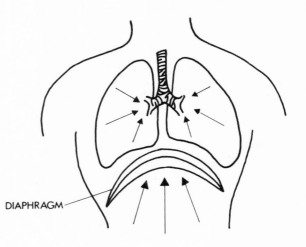

The lungs fill with air as the diaphragm descends. The diaphragm moves back up as air is exhaled.

achieves the best expansion at the base of the lungs, since the lungs themselves rest on this sheet of muscle. Because the actual exchange of oxygen and carbon dioxide takes place at the outposts, so to speak, of lung tissue. Deep complete breathing that causes air to enter the farthest recesses of the lungs is the most effective. Shallow breathing does not permit this exchange of gases, and if it is done habitually it can lead to breathlessness on mild exertion, such as walking uphill or climbing stairs. The general rule is: Breathe *in* as you stretch, extend, lift up, or move body backward; breathe *out* as you return to starting position, or to a forward or flex position. Breathe *out* when contracting the abdominal muscles.

Diaphragmatic Breathing

During *inhalation,* the diaphragm moves downward, allowing the lungs to fill up with air. The slight displacement of the abdominal contents, observed externally by a rising of the abdominal wall, differentiates a deep breath involving the diaphragm from, say, a shallow gasp, where the most obvious movement would occur near the collarbones. On *exhalation,* the diaphragm moves back up into the chest, while the lungs are emptying of air.

The term *abdominal breathing* is commonly used, but it is a misnomer — we do not and cannot breathe with the abdomen! Respiration at rest is performed most significantly

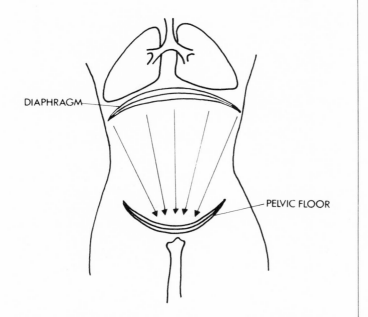

DIAPHRAGM

PELVIC FLOOR

When the pressure is increased from above, strain may be felt below.

by the diaphragm, and any "action" occurring in the abdominal area is quite passive. In fact, if the muscles of the abdomen are not relaxed and passive, then the breathing is forced up into the chest instead. This phenomenon has consequences for labor, where diaphragmatic breathing and relaxation of the abdominal wall complement each other in helping you to stay loose and to keep the breathing slow and deep.

Functions of the Diaphragm

The *diaphragm* is a broad sheet of muscle separating the chest region (with lungs and heart) from the abdominal and pelvic cavity (including the uterus). You may have never been aware of this muscle except when you have had the hiccoughs! In addition to being the major muscle of respiration, it plays a key role in many body functions, such as singing, crying, coughing, sneezing, vomiting, and elimination. It also assists the expulsive contractions of the uterus in the second stage of labor. In all these activities, the diaphragm works as an agent of pressure control. Power is provided by the abdominal muscles, which can actively contract and shorten only if a balance of air is released. This is the most efficient way of increasing the pressure in the abdominal-pelvic cavity, as can be felt in the action of playing wind instruments or blowing up inflatable toys. During pushing, the abdominal wall is drawn in, with the slow ascent of the diaphragm, as the air is exhaled against the resistance of the lips or throat. It is commonly taught that the diaphragm must be forced down like a piston and "fixed." This puts undue pressure on the pelvic floor, but fortunately the diaphragm sustains a prolonged contraction poorly.

You can well imagine how advancing pregnancy limits the action of the diaphragm. Around the eighth month, the uterus reaches its highest position abdominally, with the uppermost surface at the level of the breastbone. Due to the increasing resistance from the abdominal contents, the downward diaphragmatic movement is restricted by several inches — until the baby descends into the pelvic cavity, usually by the end of the following month. This makes breathing much easier again for the mother — although relief of these symptoms is traded for the onset of others — such as pressure on pelvic organs and blood congestion.

Learning diaphragmatic breathing will be useful for the following reasons:

- It allows for efficient expansion of the lungs and complete exchange of gases.
- Since the main vein from the lower limbs, abdomen, and pelvis passes through the diaphragm, its pumping action will improve blood circulation.
- Slow, deep rhythmical breathing is an aid to general relaxation and requires specific relaxation of the abdominal and chest muscles.
- A complete fulfilling breath feels good and does good; this is the "cleansing" or refueling breath used to start and end each labor contraction. It adds a psychological benefit: the "signing on and off" that lets you relax in the interval between contractions.
- Postpartum, this type of breathing helps to rid the body of waste products, and the effects of medication and anesthesia.
- Combined with tightening of the abdominal wall, it makes a good exercise for improving lung capacity and toning up the abdominal muscles.
- If you are confined to bed for any reason before or after delivery, a few deep complete breaths, every hour, are essential to prevent complications.

While it is possible to improve and vary chest function in many ways, the action of respiration does occur as an integrated whole. Some people find it quite difficult to learn a distinct pattern, and frequently the diaphragmatic movement is the one they cannot localize. They tend, then, to breath more with a sideways expansion of the rib cage. This difference is not important so long as you take a *complete*, deep, refreshing breath. It is the shuffling of partial air intake in the tops of the lungs, as happens in shallow upper chest breathing, that is to be discouraged.

EXERCISE 1: DIAPHRAGMATIC BREATHING

Position: Can be done in any position. When you are just starting to learn, it is easier in a comfortable supporting position, with knees bent to relax the abdominal wall. Place your hands on the abdomen, underneath the ribcage. Relax . . .

Action: Breathe in through the nose . . . let your nostrils dilate . . . and feel your abdomen "filling up with air." Then let the air escape, noticing how the abdominal wall flattens again on exhalation. Practice often throughout the day.

Note: It is easy to reverse this action, so take care that you do it correctly: Fill up as you breathe *in*; flatten as you breathe *out*. If it helps you to do it right by thinking "abdominal breathing" — then fine! If you are tense, the action will occur higher in the chest. The following progression may actually help you get started if you are still confused.

Diaphragmatic breathing

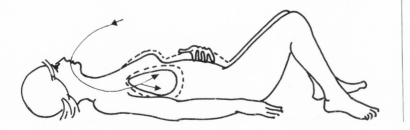

Progression: Breathe in as before, waist loose and expanding. Now, on exhaling the air, pull in your abdominal muscles and *force* it out, blowing softly yet persistently through the mouth. Keep pulling in the muscles until all the air is emptied. This way you stimulate the next intake to be more expansive, and thus with practice can improve your breathing capacity.

It is sometimes easier to learn the action by first expelling all the air completely and *then* trying for a diaphragmatic inhalation.

Warning: Breathe with moderation. Too many deep breaths in succession can cause dizziness. Deep breathing must always be kept slow, according to your own natural rhythm, never on command.

Breathing for Labor — First Stage

We have all experienced, at some time or other, a change in our breathing as an emotional reaction. When angry, excited, or afraid, we become aware of a quickened heartbeat and feel tight in the chest from interupted breathing. Normally, messages from these functions do not reach our conscious centers; the brain inhibits them so that we can direct our attention to other things. Another example is the "butterflies" in the stomach that we feel under stress. When we are in altered emotional states, the brain's inhibiting mechanism is disturbed and messages "from the gut" reach our mind.

Women in childbirth have been universally observed either to hold their breath or to accelerate their breathing spontaneously during contractions, particularly the stronger, final ones of the first stage of labor. Attending to one's breathing, then, is a way to calm the emotions and occupy the mind during labor. It is also felt that if you focus your attention on something (for example, your partner's face, not the clock's!) other than the contractions inside, they have less chance to dominate in the central exchange of the brain. It is, however, not necessary to adopt a masklike face and staring eyes or in any way to withdraw from your surroundings. Other ways to "jam the circuits" include having pleasant bodily sensations, such as those provided by massage, stroking, warmth, cold; concentrating on breathing patterns of varying rhythm; listening to music; or enjoying anything else that conditions you to feel positive mental control. When contractions are augmented by hormonal stimulants (pitocin, oxytocin) breathing skills are an essential resource. Many women use no distraction techniques at all and purposely turn their thoughts to the internal events without distress. Although some odd recommendations appear from time to time, breathing should always be easy and comfortable. As women gain more control over the circumstances under which they give birth, there will be less need for breathing patterns as a coping mechanism.

All our lives we have been effortlessly experiencing the expansion and relaxation of the chest, as the lungs inflate and deflate with our natural rhythm. Yet it is possible to localize (although not completely isolate) breathing activity in certain parts of the chest. This is a matter of emphasis, because the chest functions as a coordinated whole in normal breathing.

Breathing techniques involving the middle and upper chest are used in the Lamaze method, supposedly to lift the diaphragm off the uterus as labor advances. In the Bradley method (*Husband-Coached Childbirth*) diaphragmatic breathing is preferred as the more relaxing and physiologically advantageous form of respiration. Training in the Lamaze principles is very widespread and based on discipline, concentration, conditioning, and dissociation. A compromise has to be sought between these more artificial breathing patterns and slow or normal breathing, which some people feel does not provide a sufficient means of "control" during labor unless a woman is giving birth in the privacy and comfort of her own home. Other women are able just to "flow with the contractions," and allow their breathing to adjust physiologically to the changing intensity of the contractions. This is the best and easiest way. Some, however, use more "tools," and put in a good deal of effort, both mental and physical, to "stay on top" of the contractions with acceleration and variation of breathing. Many Lamaze mothers actually overbreathe because they are highly motivated and anxious to perform well with their breathing techniques.

The first stage of labor usually has three phases. *Early labor,* when the cervix is thinning out and dilation is getting started. Then follows the *active phase,* when the uterus works hard and consistently, gaining momentum, until the last final burst of effort (*transition*). When dilation is completed (10 cms, or 5 fingers), the first stage is over. The sequence of events is always the same, but the nature of their progression and women's experience of them vary greatly. Some labors start slowly, allowing the mother to adjust gradually to the nature of events. Others are heralded by immediate strong activity and the mother tends to be rushed along by the whole process. Guiding principles, therefore, are more valuable than a rigid set of rules.

As you near the end of the first stage, you may even feel the (perhaps premature) urge to push, which often catches you as an involuntary grunt or gasp in the throat as the uterus gets ready to expel the baby down the birth canal. Often this is the result of anxiety about one's performance or apprehension at the first sensations of rectal pressure. Brisk blowing is helpful in overcoming the desire to push with the uterus before full dilation is achieved. Blow briefly with your cheeks, not with the abdominal muscles. However, if the body is ready for you to push, the urge will be irresistible despite any breathing techniques.

Breathing is a tool that you always carry around with you; it's not something you can leave at home by mistake! The slow deep breathing already discussed will stand you in good stead for any situations of stress, excitement, or anger as well as labor. Breathing is both a mirror of the emotions and a way of modifying them and is thus intimately involved with relaxation since neither of them can be achieved without the other. Easy breathing means a relaxed body and greater comfort; if you hold your breath you will become tense.

According to yogic philosophy, the breathing must be always observed, but never controlled. The mother is seen as the vehicle for the birth and so does not control her labor. In order to flow with the process, she must center her attention and let go of the resistance in her mind as well as her body. This obviously requires self-confidence and total trust in one's body. Chanting and counting may help women center themsleves during labor. Often women invent their own techniques. It is best to be directed from within rather than by those around you. Of course, your partner and other attendants of your choosing lend great support. Praise, encouragement, and comfort measures go much further than a shot of medication.

Every birth is different, even for the same woman. You cannot know in advance how you will react to the demands of your labor. Normal breathing is clearly the most physiological. The respiratory system is very sensitive to the oxygen requirements of the body and adjustments happen automatically, as they do when you run, for example. Patterns of controlled breathing are the stalwart of most prepared childbirth programs. Taught with the best of intentions, they nevertheless interfere with relaxation (as readers can easily confirm for themselves) and lead to "performance anxiety."

*Hyper*ventilation is always a danger. This results from deep, rapid breathing, which causes too little carbon dioxide and too much oxygen in the blood. Symptoms of hyperventilation include dizziness and tingling in the lips and fingers. If carried to extremes, or combined with breath-holding, it can lead to fainting.

*Hypo*ventilation can also occur if the respiration is artificially paced. The breath has to be slow and deep enough to traverse the space between the nostrils and the air sacs of lung tissue where gaseous change occurs.

Breathing for Labor — Second Stage

As in all stages of labor, normal breathing levels should be maintained as much as possible. The coordination of breathing with abdominal muscles, which contributes to the expulsion of the baby down the birth canal, was discussed in Chapter 3, pages 52–56. Grunts and groans are preferable to holding the breath. Toward the end of second stage you will be asked to refrain from pushing so that the baby can avoid extremes of pressure and will be born gently. Contractions at the end of second stage however are more intense than at the onset. Many women gasp or pant in order to let the uterus ease the baby out of the body.

Breathing Postpartum

After delivery you need to help evacuate the waste products accumulated in the muscles and tissues from the hard work of labor, plus the effects of any medication or anesthesia. Diaphragmatic breathing hastens this process and also aids blood circulation through the pumping effect of the diaphragm on the veins returning from the legs and pelvis. The contribution of the diaphragm is important in providing intra-abdominal pressure necessary for elimination when the abdominal and pelvic floor muscles are lax. The bladder reflex is greatly diminished, since compression from the uterus is now removed and the general pressure within the abdomen is reduced.

Try to take 2 to 3 deep breaths every hour or so and always between exercises.

Persistent Coughing

A chronic chest condition is most unfortunate: it puts strain on the pelvic floor muscles and can cause or aggravate problems of sphincter weakness. The recti muscles are under greatest stress during straining with the abdominal muscles. However, by learning the proper methods of breathing and a more effective way to cough, you can learn to live more comfortably with your chest problems.

Rather than trying to jolt free any mucus in the lungs with sustained coughing, it is better to take a few minutes to mobilize and ventilate the lungs thoroughly. This technique, which expands the three key regions of the chest, is described on page 156; the same regime is used after a caesarean section. The usual type of coughing is replaced by "huffing" — a sudden retraction of the abdominal muscles on *outward* breath. Huffing is mechanically more effective and thus less tiring. You must also pull up the pelvic floor muscles as you pull in the abdominals, which avoids the sometimes alarming sensations of strain and pressure that are often felt during a regular cough.

7 | Caesarean Birth

CAESAREAN BIRTH involves the surgical delivery of the baby through the uterus and abdominal wall instead of the vagina. The lowest incidence of caesareans is around 2 to 6 percent in some countries, but at the other end of the scale the rate may be as high as 20 to 40 percent, particularly in the teaching hospitals of large urban centers. Information, understanding, and support are very necessary for couples who experience this type of delivery, largely because it tends to be overlooked that having a section is also having a baby. Discussion of caesarean birth may not be included, or may be mentioned only briefly, in childbirth preparation books and classes, yet it is the couple who have been committed to preparing for a "natural" childbirth who are often the most disappointed. In response to the needs of this growing number of parents, an organization called C/SEC (Caesareans/Support, Education, and Concern) was established in the Boston area and similar organizations can be found across the country. These groups help caesarean parents, and work to bring about changes in attitudes and policies of doctors and hospitals in order to improve the caesarean birth experience. Many books, films, and classes for planned caesareans and those aiming for a vaginal birth after caesarean (VBAC) are available today. A side effect of all this public information and education, however, is that the deplorable increase in caesareans is becoming accepted.

Indications: Sometimes a caesarean birth may be planned for in advance and is then termed "elective." Sections are most commonly done in this country because of the presence of a uterine scar from an earlier caesarean, although the belief that "once a caesarean, always a caesarean" is now changing. Frequently a caesarean birth may be anticipated but the mother is allowed a trial labor. The main reason for choosing abdominal rather than vaginal delivery is the disproportion between the size of the baby and the mother's pelvis. Sometimes the mother suffers from a general disease, such as diabetes or toxemia, which can require a caesarean birth, or there may be specific conditions within the uterus — for example, the baby or placenta lying across the cervix, separation of the placenta from the uterine wall, or prolapse of the umbilical cord — that call for a section. During labor, emergencies can arise, such as fetal distress, the failure of the uterine muscle to coordinate its action and dilate the cervix (despite a prolonged period of time), or the need to avoid a risky instrumental delivery. "Obstetrician distress" due to lack of progress in labor or anxiety about malpractice suits is also a factor. More and more physicians are routinely delivering breech babies (those presenting with the feet or buttocks) by caesarean, especially for a first-time mother. Critics of this trend feel that the poorer statistics for breech births relate more to the prematurity of the babies (as many premature babies are breech) than to the position. It may be possible, if you shop around, to find a physician who will consider a vaginal breech delivery.

Anesthesia: Local anesthesia may be given in the abdominal area. More commonly a spinal or epidural is done which provides regional anesthesia — numbness from the waist to the feet. The mother in either case is fully conscious for the event (although she does not observe the actual surgery, of course) and she can see the baby as soon as it is lifted from her body. General anesthesia is used for reasons including the necessity for speed, contra-indications to the use of spinal anesthesia, the unavailability of a specialist in this field or if mother or doctor prefer it. Since the body's reflexes are eliminated when the person is under general anesthesia, the condition of the lungs becomes of critical importance; there is a risk that the contents of the stomach may be aspirated into the lungs. This is the reason why all mothers admitted to Labor and Delivery are questioned so thoroughly with regard to what they have recently had to eat or drink; extra care will be taken during the administration of general anesthesia if it is required. Women admitted for elective caesareans must fast before surgery.

Family-centered caesarean birth: The father's right to be present at the birth, in this case taking place in the operating room, is slowly growing in acceptance. Because his mate's body is draped, he sees little more in surgery than he would in a normal birth. But the father's presence is reassuring to the mother at this stressful time and he and she share the special moment when the baby is first held up to them. The importance of this early bonding of family members is now well recognized and, since a caesarean birth is often unanticipated, the couple need each other just as much, if not more, than during a vaginal birth.

Caesarean delivery is major surgery and like others with abdominal incisions you have the discomfort of various tubes after the operation. The intravenous drip and urinary catheter from the bladder may be retained for as long as 48 hours. Fever, pain, and flatulence (gas) are common postoperative problems for which medication may be required. Itching of the skin is felt as the stitches heal. The sutures may or may not be of dissolvable material and in some hospitals metal clamps are used: the clamps and the external sutures are usually removed around the fifth or sixth day, after which you can usually go home.

Rehabilitation: It is essential for your comfort that you bridge the gap between the operating table and what is known as "early ambulation" (walking as soon as possible). Otherwise you will be hauled to your feet the following day without the transition of gradual exercise to prepare you. Pain may make it hard for you to stand with good posture; apprehension will cause you to lean "protectively" forward over the incision. The exercises are very simple and safe, and will reassure you for other activities. In most cases they are routinely given to abdominal surgery patients for their therapeutic effects, so it is ironic that caesarean mothers rarely receive this kind of postoperative care in the United States.

It *must* be emphasized that these exercises will cause *no* damage to the incision, although the first day or two it is suggested that you support the area with your hands just for your comfort. It is *essential* that you perform gentle activity with the muscles to stimulate healing. If the area is allowed to stiffen and the circulation to stagnate, the ache becomes worse and later movement is even more painful. The stitches will not pull out unless the wound is infected or the suturing was very inadequate — and in these rare instances it is much better to make this discovery as soon as possible. Exercises encourage the edges of the incision to come together, whether the incision is vertical or horizontal. The muscles are shortened and pulled in, always on the *outward* breath. Because it is difficult to inflict discomfort on yourself — even though you realize it is beneficial — your partner's encouragement and supervision are very necessary. Assistance from hospital staff is usually limited to help with early ambulation and, occasionally, the giving of a "blow bottle" to encourage deep breathing.

Caesarean Rehabilitation Exercises

EXERCISE 1: BREATHING AND HUFFING

The lungs require extra attention after surgery and if general anesthesia was used it can be expected that the lungs will collect some mucus from the slowing down of respiration. On coming out of the anesthetic, you must clear the lungs of this mucus so that chest complications are avoided.

Breathing must be done as completely as possible; all parts of the lung need to be well ventilated, although mucus tends to sink to the bases and if not removed quickly soon becomes difficult to dislodge.

Work on expanding the chest in three ways, with 2 breaths at each region. Pull *in* the abdominal muscles as you breathe *out* — and progress the muscle contraction so that you do it more strongly when the pain becomes less.

1. Diaphragmatic breathing (see page 145): Movement here may be diminished due to sensitivity of the abdominal wall. Expansion at this region is important for a complete breath, which involves the bases of the lungs.

2. Mid-chest expansion: Placing hands over the sides of the chest with gentle pressure will stimulate the sideways movement of the chest wall.

3. Upper chest expansion: Place one hand beneath the collarbones, over the breastbone, and try to move the chest underneath.

Coughing as it is generally understood is ineffective and most uncomfortable for the postoperative patient. A mother with an incision in her abdomen is so afraid that coughing will strain her stitches that at best she will just grunt feebly in the throat if asked to perform this painful feat. Huffing is much easier to do, is more effective and much less painful. Since the concept is a little strange it is a great advantage to learn it before the time an elective section is scheduled.

A *huff* is an outward breath forcefully using the diaphragm to expel air from the lungs, pulling in rather than pushing out the abdominal wall. Because the diaphragm is moving up in the chest and the abdominal muscles are shortening (instead of just tensing), the pressure is being decreased in the abdominal cavity and thus the wound is not under any strain. But unless huffing is done quickly, insufficient force is generated to dislodge any mucus. It is rather like saying "ha" but briskly and with force from the abdominal muscles. The mouth is opened wide and the jaw relaxed. Spit out any expectorate into a tissue or paper cup — don't swallow it! As a comfort measure, you may want to support the incision area with your hands or a pillow; however, be reassured again that the stitches will *not* pull out.

Huffing is also a good test to determine if there are any secretions in the lungs. If a moist rattle in the lungs is heard during this outburst of exhaled air, it indicates that mucus is present and must be removed. Don't tire yourself with huffing; once or twice is all that is usually necessary. It is better to try a round of breathing again to loosen up the chest secretions. When you have a cold or any other chest condition, you may need to work on clearing the lungs for a couple of days. If you huff and all sounds clear — then all is clear!

Breathing and huffing as just described are recommended as the most effective method of chest care for any time of life when lung secretions are increased and difficulties with respiration are present. Coughing, as commonly done, requires a brief closing of the throat and an increase of pressure within. Chronic coughing fits strain the abdominal wall and pelvic floor muscles, whereas huffing not only safeguards but actually benefits them.

EXERCISE 2: FOOT MOVEMENTS (see pages 117–118)

These are important in preventing thrombosis, particularly after anesthesia and if you are confined to bed. They can be discontinued when you start to walk around again.

Position: Legs may be out straight or loosely bent over a pillow.

Action: a) Bend and stretch your feet at the ankles. b) Make circles with your feet as the ankles, together or separately.

EXERCISE 3: LEG-BRACING

Position: Legs out straight, ankles crossed, unless you have a catheter.

Action: Tighten all the muscles in your legs, then press your knees down, tense the thigh muscles, and pull the buttocks hard together as if you were holding a coin between them. Hold for a couple of seconds and relax.

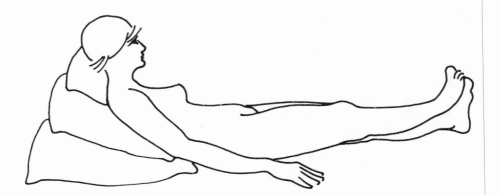

Ankles crossed, pull up the feet and brace the legs and buttocks.

Your partner can be most helpful in reminding you to take a couple of deep breaths, to wiggle your toes and bend your feet, and to tighten and relax the leg muscles frequently during the first few hours after surgery.

EXERCISE 4: BENDING AND STRAIGHTENING KNEE

Position: Lying on back, one knee bent and the other out straight.

Action: Slide the heel of the bent leg down the bed and back up to bend the knee again. Repeat with the other leg.

Bending and straightening alternate knees

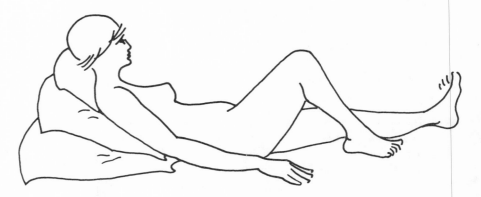

Progression: Bend one knee as you straighten the other so that you are working them together but in opposite movements.

Slide both heels down and up together at the same time.

The exercises discussed so far hasten your recovery from the anesthetic and prepare you for the effort required in first standing up after major surgery. *Before* standing, bend your knees and slowly slide your feet over to the edge of the bed. Turning with your shoulders to the same side, push up with the underneath arm and, if you wish, support the incision with your other hand for comfort. Sit for a minute or two and swing your feet up and down a few times. Brace the abdominal and buttock muscles as you gradually put the weight on your feet. Lift the upper back and stand tall; don't lean forward protectively over the incision. By retracting the abdominal muscles, you support the area with a muscular "splint," so you will not need your hands or a binder for support (although they may aid your comfort if you feel excessive anxiety, pain, or weakness). If you have done the preparatory exercises several times, this extra support should not be needed. It must be stressed again that the best support is your natural corset — the abdominal muscles.

Encouragement of activity within the abdominal cavity is essential after a caesarean delivery. Deep breathing and abdominal-wall–tightening, as already described, help to maintain intra-abdominal pressure and to relieve discomfort from air that is trapped under the diaphragm and is referred as shoulder pain. The bowel and bladder reflexes are always sluggish postpartum and are further depressed by the effects of surgery. Therefore pelvic floor contractions are important (although the baby was not born vaginally) to help stimulate activity within the pelvic cavity.

The greatest problem postpartum is the formation and retention of gas within the intestines. The peak of this discomfort is reached around the second or third postoperative day, when the natural wave of intestinal movement (peristalsis) recurs. The abdomen can become bloated and the movement of the gas within the intestines quite visible. Exercises that provide gentle movement and compression of the abdominal contents are essential to prevent the pain and distress that otherwise occur. Some relief from these symptoms can be obtained by lying on the left side, with your knees bent, so that gravity encourages the natural progress of the gas through the intestines, and gently kneading the abdominal wall.

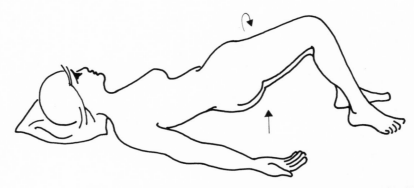

Bridge and twist the hips — first to the right, then to the left — and lower.

EXERCISE 5: PELVIC-ROCKING

Position: Lying on your back or side, with knees bent.

Action: This is the same movement as described on page 68, but in this case it is done with the intent to stimulate sluggish intestinal activity rather than to strengthen the muscles that control the pelvic tilt.

Gently rock the pelvis back and forth, using your abdominal and buttock muscles.

EXERCISE 6: BRIDGE AND TWIST

Position: Lying on your back with knees bent, with just one pillow.

Action: Contract your buttocks and abdominal muscles and raise your hips a few inches off the bed. Maintain this elevated position as you twist your hips to the right and then to the left. Lower the buttocks back to the bed and relax. Keep the sphincters and buttocks tightly closed during these movements.

EXERCISE 7: REACH TO THE KNEES

Position: Half-lying with the back of the bed raised or several pillows behind your head and shoulders.

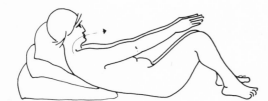

Action: Tuck your chin in and tilt your pelvis back. Lean forward to reach toward your knees with your hands. Lower your head and shoulders back on the pillow and relax.

It is important to breathe in deeply before starting, and as you move forward to breathe out while pulling in the abdominal muscles. For additional comfort you may wish to support the incision area with your hands.

Before leaving the hospital, check for separation of the recti muscles (see pages 60–63) and then progress at your own pace with the exercises recommended for the normal postpartum. Especially avoid lifting, straining, undue exertion, and poor body mechanics (see Chapter 4).

Comfort Measures

When *feeding your baby,* place a pillow between him or her and your incision or lie on your side and nurse the baby from that position. You can also try placing the baby against you so that the head is at the breast but the feet in the opposite direction, that is, behind your shoulder.

Take it easy. This does not mean refrain from the rehabilitation exercises if you feel tired; they are the very ones that will hasten your recovery and ease your discomfort. But you will experience much fatigue since you have had not only a baby but surgery as well. So relaxation sessions must not be neglected. Sometimes caesarean mothers are warned against climbing stairs or even riding in a car! Unfortunately, this well-intended advice would prolong their convalescence by making them reluctant to perform the mildest activity. Stairs are much more tiring than regular walking, because they demand muscle work against gravity. You must take them very slowly, one at a time, to avoid exhaustion. Do not hold your breath; use your legs to propel your body upward. (See page 107 for the correct way to go up and down stairs.) Long drives can also be very fatiguing at this time. For your comfort in the car, place a pillow or sanitary pad between you and the seatbelt while there is tenderness around the incision (see page 92). Try to always have someone with you for the first week at home and avoid doing any unnecessary chores so that you can recover as quickly as possible.

Summaries of Essential Exercises

The posture checklist and following three summary pages are designed to be removed from the book for handy reference.

Posture Checklist

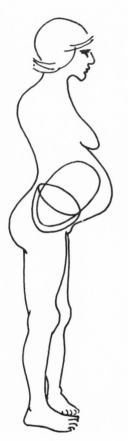

Incorrect Posture	To correct posture:
HEAD	
If neck sags, chin pokes forward, and whole body slumps.	Straighten neck, tuck chin in, so body lines up.
SHOULDERS AND CHEST	
Slouching cramps the rib cage and makes breathing difficult. Arms turn in.	Lift up through rib cage and pull back shoulder girdle. Roll arms out.
ABDOMEN AND BUTTOCKS	
Slack muscles = hollow-back. Pelvis tilts forward.	Contract abdominals to flatten back. Tuck buttocks under and tilt pelvis back.
KNEES	
Pressed back strains joints, pushes pelvis forward.	Bend to ease body weight over feet.
FEET	
Weight on inner borders strains arches.	Distribute body weight through center of each foot.

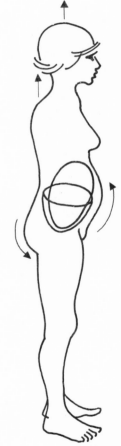

From *Essential Exercises for the Childbearing Year*, © 1976 Elizabeth Noble, Houghton Mifflin Company

Summary of Essential Prenatal Exercises

Do each exercise twice at first, progressing at your own pace to 5 times. The sequence can be repeated in reverse order. Relax and breathe deeply between each exercise.

1. Deep breathing with Abdominal-Wall–Tightening on outward breath (page 66).

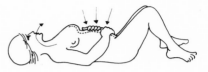

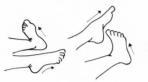

2. Foot Exercises: stretch, bend, and rotate (page 118).

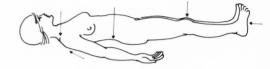

3. Stretch out the Kinks: on the bed, against wall (page 115).

4. Pelvic Floor: 4 exercises (pages 41–44)

5. Pelvic-Tilting: various positions (page 68).

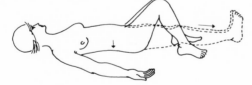

6. Leg-Sliding (page 74).

7. Straight Curl-up (page 76).

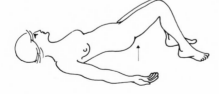

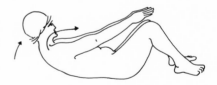

8. Bridging (page 116).

9. Diagonal Curl-up (page 78).

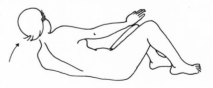

When *standing up,* roll over onto the knees and push arm with the arms. When rising from the floor, go on to one knee and straighten legs to stand (page 106).

10. *Posture Check:* (page 161).

Relaxation session: Twenty minutes' complete tension release in any position of comfort twice daily.

Summary of Essential Postpartum Exercises

Commence within 24 hours; repeat each exercise twice to start, progressing at your own pace through the phases. Relax and breathe deeply between each exercise. The sequence can be repeated in reverse order. Do the exercises at least twice daily.

Phase I

1. Deep breathing with Abdominal-Wall–Tightening on outward breath (page 66).

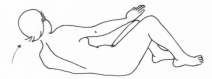

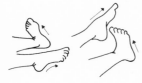

2. Foot Exercises: bend, stretch, and rotate (page 118). Continue until walking around.

3. Stretch out the Kinks (page 115).

4. Pelvic Floor Contractions (page 41).

5. Pelvic-Tilting: (page 68).

Before standing: Sit with legs over bed for a few minutes and swing the feet. Brace abdominals, buttocks, and pelvic floor when upright and walking around at first.

Posture check: (page 161).

Relaxation: Lying on the front (page 92). Twice daily, at least half an hour.

Add Phase II

6. Leg-Sliding (page 74).

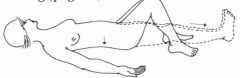

7. Bridging (page 116).

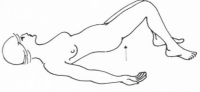

Add Phase III

Check for separation of the recti muscles after third day (page 61). Check stopping and starting urine flow (page 43).

8. Straight Curl-up (page 76).

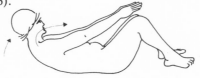

9. Diagonal Curl-up (page 78).

Phase IV

Progressive abdominal exercises (pages 79–81).

Summary of Essential Exercises Following Caesarean Birth

Commence as soon as you recover from the anesthetic. Do each exercise twice to start, progressing at your own pace through the phases. Relax and breathe deeply between each exercise. The sequence can be repeated in reverse order.

Phase I

1. Breathing Exercises: Upper chest, mid-chest, diaphragmatic with abdominal-wall–tightening (pages 66, 153).

2. Huffing (page 153). These two are very important if general anesthesia was used.

3. Foot Exercises: bend, stretch, rotate (page 118).

4. Leg-Bracing: tense and relax legs (page 157). Continue these for as long as you are confined to bed.

Phase II

5. Bending and Straightening Alternate Knee (page 156).

6. Pelvic-Rocking (page 159). Combine with pelvic floor contractions.

Before standing: Bend knees; use arms to turn toward edge of bed. Sit first and swing feet a few times. Brace abdominal muscles as you stand upright.
Posture check: (page 161).

Add Phase III

7. Bridge and Twist (page 158).

8. Reach to the Knees (page 158).

Add Phase IV

Check for separation of the recti muscles (page 61). Check stopping and starting the urine flow (page 43).

9. Straight Curl-up (page 76).

10. Leg-Sliding (page 74).

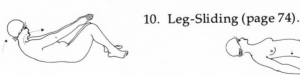

11. Diagonal Curl-up (page 78).

12. Relaxation on front when comfort permits. (page 92).

Phase V

Progressive abdominal exercises (pages 79–81).

From *Essential Exercises for the Childbearing Year,* © 1976 Elizabeth Noble, Houghton Mifflin Company

Anderson, Bob. *Stretching*. Bolinas, California: Shelter Publications, 1980. An excellent and well-illustrated book for everyone. Provides simplifications of many yoga positions.

Arms, Suzanne. *A Season to Be Born*. New York: Harper & Row, 1973. Superb photographs of a mother's experience of pregnancy and birth.

Arms, Suzanne. *Immaculate Deception*. Boston: Houghton Mifflin Co., 1975. Describes how hospitals complicate childbirth, compares childbirth practices in other countries, presents a strong argument for home birth.

Ballentine, R. *Diet and Nutrition*. Honesdale, Pennsylvania: Himalayan International Institute, 1978. A very readable overview of nutrition covering both Eastern and Western views.

Bean, Constance. *Labor and Delivery: An Observer's Diary*. New York: Doubleday & Co., 1977. Insights into hospital birth experiences.

Bean, Constance. *Methods of Childbirth*. New York: Doubleday & Co., 1972. Excellent general guide for choosing hospital, doctor, childbirth classes, drugs, etc. Encourages consumers to exercise their options as adults rather than patients.

Benson, Herbert, M.D. *The Relaxation Response*. New York: William Morrow, 1975. A recent study showing how meditation techniques such as transcendental meditation benefit the body. For lay readers.

Benson, Ralph. *Handbook of Obstetrics and Gynecology*, 5th edition. Los Altos, California: Lange Medical Publications, 1974. Although intended for medical professionals, this concise, clearly illustrated text is highly recommended. Excellent organization of material makes this a handy reference; includes details of home birth, caesarean section.

Bing, Elisabeth. *The Adventure of Birth*. New York: Ace, 1970. Forty-one couples describe their personal experiences in hospitals to this famous Lamaze instructor.

Bing, Elisabeth, and Libby Colman. *Making Love During Pregnancy*. New York: Bantam Books, 1977. A sensitive and beautifully illustrated book.

Bradley, R., M.D. *Husband-Coached Childbirth*. New York: Harper & Row, 1974. This is a family-centered approach which encourages couples to find their own style in labor. Relaxation emphasized more than breathing techniques.

Brewer, Gail Storza, with Tom Brewer, M.D., consultant. *What Every Pregnant Woman Should Know: The Truth About Drugs and Diet in Pregnancy*. New York: Random House, 1977; Baltimore, Maryland: Penguin, 1979. A discussion of harmful dietary advice, and the importance of good nutrition in preventing toxemia.

Brewer, Gail Storza, ed. *The Pregnancy After 30 Workbook*. Emmaus, Pennsylvania: Rodale Press, 1979. An excellent general guide.

Boston Women's Health Book Collective. *Our Bodies, Ourselves*, 2nd edition. New York: Simon & Schuster, 1976. Comprehensive book on womanhood and self-help. Excellent bibliographies.

References and Suggested Reading

Colman, Arthur, M.D., and Libby Colman, Ph.D. *Pregnancy, the Psychological Experience.* New York: Herder & Herder, 1971. Absorbing book which deals with the range of feelings experienced by both parents.

Cooper, Kenneth H., M.D., M.P.H. *The New Aerobics.* New York: Bantam, 1970. Graded physical fitness program for general activities such as running, swimming, and bicycling.

Consumers' Union. *The Medicine Show,* Revised Edition. New York: Pantheon Books, Random House, 1974. A critical discussion of common drugstore products with a chapter on drugs in pregnancy.

Deutsch, Ronald M. *The Key to Feminine Response in Marriage.* New York: Ballantine, 1968. The unfortunate title obscures the excellent presentation of the research of Kegel and Masters and Johnson and the importance of pelvic floor control.

"Frankly Speaking: A Pamphlet for Caesarean Couples," 2nd ed. C/SEC (15 Maynard Road, Dedham, Massachusetts 02026), 1978.

Gaskin, Ina May. *Spiritual Midwifery.* Summertown, Tennessee: The Book Publishing Company, 1978. Accounts of many alternative births plus a good technical reference section.

Graedon, Joe. *The People's Pharmacy: A Guide to Prescription Drugs, Home Remedies, and Over the Counter Medications.* New York: St. Martin's Press, 1976. A good family reference discussing the effects and side effects of pharmaceutical items.

Haire, Doris B., D.M.S. *The Cultural Warping of Childbirth: A Special Report on U.S. Obstetrics.* ICEA Bookcenter (P.O. Box 20048, Minneapolis, Minnesota 55426), 1972. Shows how poorly the U.S. measures up when compared with other countries.

Hazell, Lester. *Commonsense Childbirth.* New York: Tower, 1975. An excellent general book; includes discussion of home birth and breast-feeding.

Jacobson, Edmund. *How to Relax and Have Your Baby.* New York: McGraw-Hill, 1965. A classic by one of the first physicians to work with relaxation.

Kendall, Henry, Florence Kendall, and Dorothy Boynton. *Posture and Pain.* Baltimore: Williams & Wilkins, 1952. Written for health professionals, but contains clear descriptions and illustrations of problems with body mechanics with appropriate exercises.

Kitzinger, Sheila. *The Experience of Childbirth,* 3rd edition. Great Britain: G. Nichols & Co., 1974. British author emphasizes harmony of the body with feelings and emotions; discusses importance of the pelvic floor release during birth.

Kitzinger, Sheila. *Giving Birth: The Parents' Experience of Childbirth.* New York: Taplinger, 1971. A collection of personal accounts expressing the individuality and range of experiences.

Kraus, Hans, M.D. *Backache, Stress and Tension: Their Cause, Prevention and Treatment.* New York: Pocket Books, 1969. Specialist in physical medicine discusses the role of preventive exercise with basic self-tests and corrective exercise schemes.

Lang, Raven. *Birth Book*. Palo Alto, California: Genesis Press, 1972. Personal descriptions of home births; exceptional photographs.

Leboyer, Frederick. *Inner Beauty, Inner Light: Yoga for Pregnant Women*. New York: Alfred Knopf, 1977. A poetic book with emphasis on the natural and spiritual aspects of pregnancy and birth.

Masters, William H., and Virginia E. Johnson. *Human Sexual Response*. Boston: Little Brown, 1966. The scientific landmark that made knowledge of human sexuality objective and debunked many myths.

Melzack, Ronald. *The Puzzle of Pain*. New York: Basic Books, 1973 (both hardcover and paperback). A technical work dealing with the gate control theory.

Milinaire, Caterine. *Birth*. New York: Harmony Books, 1974. Assortment of information presented in a readable, personable style. Accounts of different births and life styles.

Mitchell, Laura. *Simple Relaxation*. New York: Atheneum, 1979. A unique guide based on physiological principles.

Mitchell, Laura, and Barbara Dale. *Simple Movement: The Why and How of Exercise*. London: John Murray, 1981. A readable text explaining how the body works, with a total exercise program.

Montagu, Ashley. *Touching: The Human Significance of the Skin*. New York: Perennial Library, Harper & Row, 1971. Fascinating evaluation of our need for physical contact; draws on anthropological and animal studies to emphasize importance of breast-feeding, rocking, cradles, etc.

Parfitt, Rebecca. *The Birth Primer. A Source of Traditional and Alternative Methods in Labor and Delivery*. Philadelphia: Running Press, 1977.

Rozdilsky, M., and B. Banet. *What Now? A Handbook for New Parents*. New York: Scribner, 1975.

Shepro, David, Ph.D., and Howard Knuttgen, Ph.D. *Complete Conditioning: The No-Nonsense Guide to Fitness and Good Health*. Philippines: Addison-Wesley, 1976. Emphasizes cardiovascular fitness, with information on exercise, nutrition, weight control, and all kinds of fads and gadgets.

Ward, Charlotte, and Fred Ward. *The Home Birth Book*. Washington, D.C.: New Perspectives, Inscape Publishers, 1976. Various authors present the different dimensions of home birth. Shows that this growing trend is spreading to all social groups.

White, Gregory, M.D. *Emergency Childbirth*. Franklin Park, Illinois: Police Training Foundation, 1958. Essential if planning a nonhospital birth. Author's low-key approach, with the view that in over 95 percent of such cases the "simple tasks could be performed by any bright eight-year-old," reassure the reader's confidence in her body and the processes of nature.

White, John, and James Fadiman, eds. *Relax: How You Can Feel Better, Reduce Stress and Overcome Tension*. New York: Dell Publishing Co.: 1976. Extensive overview of all methods with excerpts from different authors.

Resources

The American Academy of Husband-Coached Childbirth, P.O. Box 5224, Sherman Oaks, California 91413 (Bradley method).

American College of Home Obstetrics, % Gregory White, M.D., 2821 Rose Street, Franklin Park, Illinois 60131.

The American College of Nurse-Midwives, 1012 14th Street N.W., Washington, D.C. 20005.

American Foundation for Maternal and Child Health, Inc., 30 Beekman Place, New York, New York 10022.

American Society of Psychoprophylaxis in Obstetrics (ASPO), 1411 K Street N.W., Suite 200, Washington, D.C. 20005 (Lamaze method).

Association for Childbirth at Home International, Box 1219, Cerritos, California 90701.

Council of Childbirth Education Specialists, Inc. (C/CES), 168 West 86th Street, New York, New York 10024 (The Lamaze method of prepared childbirth).

Health Technology Associates, Ltd., 70 Spruce Street, Burlington, Vermont 05401 (Resources, referrals, and counseling on pelvic floor function and female ejaculation).

Holistic Childbirth Institute, 1627 Tenth Ave., San Francisco, California 94112.

Home Oriented Maternity Experience (HOME), 511 New York Ave., Takoma Park, Washington, D.C. 20012.

Informed Homebirth, 1811 Burns Street, Detroit, Michigan 48214.

International Childbirth Education Association (ICEA), P.O. Box 20048, Minneapolis, Minnesota 55420 (Provides information on all aspects of childbirth and parenting. ICEA Bookcenter specializes in books on birth, parenting, and child development).

La Leche League International, 9616 Minneapolis Ave., Franklin Park, Illinois 60131 (Breast-feeding).

Maternity Center Association, 48 East Ninety-second Street, New York, New York 10028.

National Association of Parents and Professionals for Safe Alternatives in Childbirth (NAPPSAC), P.O. Box 267, Marble Hill, Missouri 63764.

National Organization of Mothers of Twins Clubs, 5402 Amberwood Lane, Rockville, Maryland 20853 (Write for information on U.S. state and local chapters. The national group publishes "Notebook," a quarterly publication, and a bibliography of booklets on twin care by local chapters. Godmothers, grandmothers, and legal guardians of multiples are also eligible to join.)

Obstetrics and Gynecology Section, American Physical Therapy Association, 1156 15th Street N.W., Washington, D.C. 20005.

Polymorph Films, 118 South Street, Boston, Massachusetts 02111 (*Essential Exercises for the Childbearing Year* and other films on birth, child care, and parenting available for purchase or rental).

Read Natural Childbirth Foundation, 13301 Eliseo Drive, Suite 102, Greenbrae, California 94904 (The Grantly Dick-Read method of prepared childbirth).

Sex Information and Education Council of the U.S. (SIECUS), 1855 Broadway, New York, New York 10010.

Society for the Protection of the Unborn Through Nutrition, Suite 603, 17 North Wabash Ave., Chicago, Illinois 60602.

Vaginal Birth After Caesarean (VBAC), 10 Great Plain Terrace, Needham, Massachusetts 02192 (For information on VBAC, send a self-addressed, stamped envelope and $1 to Nancy Cohen at the above address.)

Index